Heart Failure

Editors

JENNIFER KITCHENS
LENORA MAZE

CRITICAL CARE NURSING CLINICS OF NORTH AMERICA

www.ccnursing.theclinics.com

Consulting Editor
JAN FOSTER

December 2015 • Volume 27 • Number 4

ELSEVIER

1600 John F. Kennedy Boulevard ● Suite 1800 ● Philadelphia, Pennsylvania, 19103-2899

http://www.theclinics.com

CRITICAL CARE NURSING CLINICS OF NORTH AMERICA Volume 27, Number 4
December 2015 ISSN 0899-5885, ISBN-13: 978-0-323-40242-2

Editor: Kerry Holland
Developmental Editor: Colleen Viola

Critical Care Nursing Clinics of North America (ISSN 0899-5885) is published quarterly by Elsevier Inc., 360 Park Avenue South, New York, NY 10010-1710. Months of issue are March, June, September, and December. Business and Editorial Offices: 1600 John F. Kennedy Blvd., Suite 1800, Philadelphia, PA 19103-2899. Periodicals postage paid at New York, NY and additional mailing offices. Subscription prices are $150.00 per year for US individuals, $328.00 per year for US institutions, $80.00 per year for US students and residents, $200.00 per year for Canadian individuals, $412.00 per year for Canadian institutions, $230.00 per year for international individuals, $412.00 per year for international institutions and $115.00 per year for Canadian and international students/residents. To receive student/resident rate, orders must be accompanied by name of affiliated institution, data of term, and the *signature* of program/residency coordinator on institution letterhead. Orders will be billed at individual rate until proof of status is received. Foreign air speed delivery is included in all *Clinics* subscription prices. All prices are subject to change without notice. **POSTMASTER:** Send address changes to *Critical Care Nursing Clinics of North America*, Elsevier Health Sciences Division, Subscription Customer Service, 3251 Riverport Lane, Maryland Heights, MO 63043. **Customer Service: 1-800-654-2452 (US and Canada); 314-447-8871 (outside US and Canada). Fax: 314-447-8029. E-mail:** JournalsCustomerService-usa@elsevier.com **(for print support) and** JournalsOnlineSupport-usa@elsevier.com **(for online support).**

Reprints. For copies of 100 or more of articles in this publication, please contact the Commercial Reprints Department, Elsevier Inc., 360 Park Avenue South, New York, New York, 10010-1710; Tel.: 212-633-3874, Fax: 212-633-3820, and E-mail: reprints@elsevier.com.

Critical Care Nursing Clinics of North America is covered in *MEDLINE/PubMed (Index Medicus), International Nursing Index, Nursing Citation Index, Cumulative Index to Nursing and Allied Health Literature, and RNdex Top 100.*

Contributors

CONSULTING EDITOR

JAN FOSTER, PhD, APRN, CNS
Formerly, Associate Professor, College of Nursing, Texas Woman's University, Houston; Currently, President, Nursing Inquiry and Intervention Inc., The Woodlands, Texas

EDITORS

JENNIFER KITCHENS, MSN, RN, ACNS-BC, CVRN
Clinical Nurse Specialist, Acuity Adaptable, Risk Management, Eskenazi Health, Indianapolis, Indiana

LENORA MAZE, MSN, RN, CNRN
Clinical Nurse Specialist, Critical Care and Neuroscience, Risk Management, Eskenazi Health, Indianapolis, Indiana

AUTHORS

WINDY ALONSO, MS, RN
Research Assistant and Doctoral Student, The Pennsylvania State University College of Nursing, Hershey, Pennsylvania

JONATHAN AULD, MS, MA, RN, CNL
PhD Student, School of Nursing and Knight Cardiovascular Institute, Oregon Health and Science University, Portland, Oregon

CINDY BITHER, MSN, ANP-C, ACNP-C, CHFN
Chief Nurse Practitioner, Advanced Heart Failure Program, Medstar Washington Hospital Center, Washington, DC

DIANE DOTY, MS, BSN, RN, CCRN, CCNS
Clinical Nurse Specialist, Community Health Network, Indianapolis, Indiana

JAMES H. FULLER, PharmD
President, Indianapolis Coalition for Patient Safety, Inc, Indianapolis, Indiana

DANA HARRIS, BSN, RN, CHFN
Carolinas Healthcare System, Sanger Heart and Vascular Institute, Charlotte, North Carolina

JUDITH E. HUPCEY, EdD, CRNP, FAAN
Professor of Nursing, The Pennsylvania State University College of Nursing, Hershey, Pennsylvania

JOANNA KINGERY, PharmD
Director, Statewide Advanced Heart Care, Indiana University Health, Indianapolis, Indiana

JENNIFER KITCHENS, MSN, RN, ACNS-BC, CVRN
Clinical Nurse Specialist, Acuity Adaptable, Risk Management, Eskenazi Health, Indianapolis, Indiana

LISA KITKO, PhD, RN
Assistant Professor of Nursing, The Pennsylvania State University College of Nursing, University Park, Pennsylvania

JANET A. KLOOS, RN, PhD, MSN, CCNS, CCRN
Clinical Nurse Specialist, University Hospitals Case Medical Center, Harrington Heart and Vascular Institute, Cleveland, Ohio

CHRISTOPHER S. LEE, PhD, RN, FAHA, FAAN
Associate Professor, School of Nursing and Knight Cardiovascular Institute, Oregon Health and Science University, Portland, Oregon

BRENDA McCULLOCH, RN, MSN
Cardiovascular Clinical Nurse Specialist, Sutter Medical Center, Sacramento, California

BARBARA McLEAN, MN, RN, CCNS-BC, NP-BC, CCRN, FCCM
Consultant in Critical Care; Clinical Specialist, Division of Critical Care, Grady Health System, Atlanta, Georgia

KRISTIN MONZA, MSN, RN, CHFN
Carolinas Healthcare System, Sanger Heart and Vascular Institute, Charlotte, North Carolina

ASHLEY MOORE-GIBBS, MSN, AGPCNP-BC, CHFN
Nurse Practitioner, Advanced Heart Failure Program, Medstar Washington Hospital Center, Washington, DC

ARIF NAZIR, MD, FACP
Associate Professor of Clinical Medicine, Eskenazi Health, Indiana University School of Medicine, Indianapolis, Indiana

KIMBERLY A. NELSON, DNP, RN-BC, ACNS-BC, CHFN, CCPC, CCRP, RDCS
Nurse Clinician, Virginia Commonwealth University Medical Center, Richmond, Virginia

CARMEN SHAW, MSN, RN-BC
Carolinas Healthcare System, Sanger Heart and Vascular Institute, Charlotte, North Carolina

DEBORAH A. TAYLOR, PharmD
Clinical Pharmacist, Department of Pharmacy and Clinical Nutrition, Grady Health System, Atlanta, Georgia

ROBIN J. TRUPP, PhD, RN, ACNP-BC, CHFN, FAHA
Adjunct Assistant Clinical Professor, University of Illinois at Chicago, College of Nursing, Chicago, Illinois

Contents

Heart Failure: A Primer   413

Christopher S. Lee and Jonathan Auld

>Heart failure is a complex and multisystem clinical syndrome that results from impaired ventricular contractility and/or relaxation. Hypertension, diabetes mellitus, and coronary artery disease are common antecedents to heart failure. The main pathogenic mechanisms involved in heart failure include sympathetic nervous and renin-angiotensin-aldosterone system activation, as well as inflammation. A detailed history and physical examination and additional diagnostic tests may be needed to diagnose heart failure. Most treatment strategies target neurohormonal systems. Non-pharmacologic interventions and effective engagement in self-care are also important in overall heart failure management. Therapeutic strategies are geared toward prolonging life and optimizing quality of life.

Heart Failure and Atrial Fibrillation   427

Brenda McCulloch

>Atrial fibrillation is commonly experienced by patients with heart failure, and as the heart failure progresses and worsens, the more likely the patient is to develop atrial fibrillation. Several factors play into this, including common risk factors, such as advanced age, hypertension, and ischemic or valvular heart disease. Treatment is aimed at anticoagulation, to prevent thromboembolic stroke, and rate control to prevent further hemodynamic compromise. Rhythm control may be beneficial for many patients, and this can be accomplished through the use of antiarrhythmic medications, cardioversion, and/or ablation.

Hypertensive Crisis: A Review of Pathophysiology and Treatment   439

Deborah A. Taylor

>Hypertensive crisis presents as hypertensive urgency or hypertensive emergency, the differences being the presence or absence of target organ damage (TOD) and the type of treatment the patient will receive. Patients with hypertensive urgency do not express TOD, which is seen only in hypertensive emergencies and can involve the heart, kidneys, or brain. Recognition of hypertensive crisis at initial assessment is crucial. An important first step is to obtain a full medical and medication history to be used as a guide for treatment. Proper and effective treatment of hypertensive urgency or emergency involves appropriate use of specific agents based on knowledge of any comorbid disease state.

In critically ill patients with circulatory shock, the role of the left ventricle has long been appreciated and the object of measurement and therapeutic targeting. The right ventricle is often under-appreciated, and dysfunction may be overlooked. Generally, the right ventricle operates passively to support the ejection of the left ventricular diastolic volume. A loss of right ventricular wall compliance secondary to pulmonary pressures may result in an alteration in the normal pressure-volume relationship, ultimately affecting the stroke volume and cardiac output. Traditional right heart filling indices may increase because of decreasing compliance, further complicating the picture. The pathophysiology of pulmonary vascular dysfunction in acute respiratory distress syndrome combined with the effects of a mean airway pressure strategy may create an acute cor pulmonale.

Cardiotoxicity is a broad term that refers to the negative effects of toxic substances on the heart. Cancer drugs can cause cardiotoxicity by effects on heart cells, thromboembolic events, and/or hypertension that can lead to heart failure. Rheumatoid arthritis biologics may interfere with ischemic preconditioning and cause/worsen heart failure. Long-term and heavy alcohol use can result in oxidative stress, apoptosis, and decreased contractile protein function. Cocaine use results in sympathetic nervous system stimulation of heart and smooth muscle cells and leads to cardiotoxicity and evolution of heart failure. The definition of cardiotoxicity is likely to evolve along with knowledge about detecting subclinical myocardial injury.

Acute pericarditis occurs most frequently after a viral attack. Other causes are autoimmune conditions, infection, chest trauma, cardiac surgery, or cardiac procedure. The presenting symptom is retrosternal chest pain. A pericardial rub is characteristic. Diffuse upward sloping ST segments are found with electrocardiogram. Pericardial effusions may be demonstrated with an echocardiogram. High-dose nonsteroidal antiinflammatory medications are the primary treatment. Adding colchicine reduces recurrence. It responds well to pharmacologic therapy within 1 to 2 weeks. Monitoring for complications is essential. The most serious complication is cardiac tamponade. For this, prompt diagnosis and treatment can be life-saving.

High-output heart failure is not seen as commonly as low-output heart failure, and some of the typical guideline recommendations may not benefit patients with high-output failure. High-output failure is caused by several diseases, including thyrotoxicosis and beriberi, highlighted in this article. Thyrotoxicosis, caused by excessive thyroid hormone production, has profound hemodynamic effects. Wet beriberi, predominately affecting the cardiovascular system, is caused by severe thiamine deficiency, most commonly seen in patients with chronic alcoholism or poor nutrition from other causes. Prompt recognition of these infrequently seen syndromes is essential. This article outlines the medical treatment and nursing care needed to return these patients to a normal state.

Sleep deprivation occurs for many reasons but, when chronic in nature, has many consequences for optimal health and performance. Despite its high prevalence, sleep-disordered breathing is underrecognized and undertreated. This is especially true in the setting of heart failure, where sleep-disordered breathing affects more than 50% of patients. Although the optimal strategy to identify patients is currently unknown, concerted and consistent efforts to support early recognition, diagnosis, and subsequent treatment should be encouraged. Optimization of guideline-directed medical therapy and concurrent treatment of sleep-disordered breathing are necessary to improve outcomes in this complex high-risk population.

Indianapolis Coalition for Patient Safety, Inc engaged a citywide effort to reduce hospital readmissions of patients diagnosed with heart failure within 30 days of discharge. An innovative collaboration among interdisciplinary representatives of hospitals, skilled nursing facilities, and home care agencies resulted in a reduction in readmissions for patients with heart failure.

Today's health care systems are faced with challenges to transform health care delivery and provide quality and valued services for the heart failure population. These challenges require collaboration and the development of strategic processes that will redefine best practices. Implementing a multidimensional nurse navigator transition program is one approach to facilitating cross-continuum of care. Such a program has been proven to significantly reduce 30-day all-cause hospital readmissions, enhance self-management skills, and improve follow-up compliance. This transitional care model can be used to address the needs of all patients with chronic conditions.

Mechanical circulatory support (MCS) devices offer advanced heart failure patients a potential long-term solution. MCS devices implantation is increasing related to the increased volume of heart failure patients, the shortfall of suitable donors, and the advanced technology and smaller size of the devices. To ensure a successful outcome, some key elements must be taken into consideration and managed: patient selection, preoperative preparation, intraoperative care, postoperative care, and posthospital education. The ultimate success of an MCS implantation relies on a multidisciplinary approach and excellent patient/caregiver education in each phase of hospitalization.

Heart transplantation is a recommended and curative treatment option for patients with advanced heart failure symptoms despite receiving optimal medical and device therapy. The availability of donor organs limits the number of patients able to receive a heart transplant. The overall outcome of patients able to receive a heart transplant is determined by the successful delivery of essential nursing care. Understanding the specific interventions and therapies unique to this patient population is critical to their care. This article reviews considerations for the intensive care unit clinician in the management of heart transplant patients in this setting.

The number of patients with heart failure is growing; the associated morbidity and mortality remains dismal. Advance care planning, end-of-life conversations, and palliative care referrals are appropriate, but do not occur regularly. Palliative care focuses on patients and families from diagnosis, to hospice, death, and bereavement. It is delivered as basic palliative care by all providers and by specialty-certified palliative care specialists. Nurses are instrumental in initiating referrals to the specialized palliative care team as the patient's needs become too complex or the disease progresses and the patient approaches the end of life.

CRITICAL CARE NURSING CLINICS OF NORTH AMERICA

THE CLINICS ARE AVAILABLE ONLINE!
Access your subscription at:
www.theclinics.com

Preface

Heart Failure

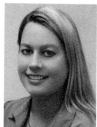
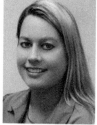

Jennifer Kitchens, MSN, RN, ACNS-BC, CVRN   Lenora Maze, MSN, RN, CNRN
Editors

The cost impact of heart failure in the critical care environment and health care system, as a whole, is significant. Heart failure is the only cardiovascular disease that is increasing. There are 6.5 million hospital days a year and nearly $40 billion dollars in yearly health care costs attributed to heart failure in the United States. Over $2.9 billion dollars is spent annually on the pharmaceutical management of heart failure in the United States. There are more Medicare monies spent for diagnosing and treating heart failure than any other diagnosis-related group. This diagnosis is the leading cause of hospitalization for patients who are 65 years of age and older. There is a 24% 30-day hospital readmission rate for this diagnosis, which leads to financial implications for health care systems.

The human cost is also significant. Less than half of Americans diagnosed with heart failure survive more than 5 years. The ongoing health care needs and cost of this chronic disease take a significant toll on patients' finances, time, and quality of life. Few health care providers in the critical care environment are not affected by heart failure on a routine basis. Caring for these patients and their families is both a challenging and yet a rewarding experience. Critical care nurses can benefit from expanded knowledge of heart failure strategies and interventions to appropriately manage patient care throughout the trajectory of this illness. This issue provides critical care nurses with a comprehensive heart failure review, which is essential given the dynamic health and critical care environments. We would like to thank each of the authors for sharing their expertise with nurses who care for patients with heart failure in the critical care setting.

Crit Care Nurs Clin N Am 27 (2015) xi–xii
http://dx.doi.org/10.1016/j.cnc.2015.09.001
0899-5885/15/$ – see front matter © 2015 Published by Elsevier Inc.

ccnursing.theclinics.com

We found both the topics and the content of various aspects of heart failure care to be exceptional and hope that you agree.

Jennifer Kitchens, MSN, RN, ACNS-BC, CVRN
Clinical Nurse Specialist
Acuity Adaptable
Risk Management
Eskenazi Health
720 Eskenazi Avenue
Indianapolis, IN 46202, USA

Lenora Maze, MSN, RN, CNRN
Clinical Nurse Specialist
Critical Care and Neuroscience
Risk Management
Eskenazi Health
720 Eskenazi Avenue
Indianapolis, IN 46202, USA

E-mail addresses:
jennifer.kitchens@eskenazihealth.edu (J. Kitchens)
lenora.maze@eskenazihealth.edu (L. Maze)

Heart Failure: A Primer

Christopher S. Lee, PhD, RN*, Jonathan Auld, MS, MA, RN, CNL

KEYWORDS

- Heart failure • Congestive heart failure • Pathophysiology • Self-management

KEY POINTS

- Heart failure is a clinical syndrome that results from impaired ventricular contractility and/or relaxation.
- Although many cases of heart failure are idiopathic, hypertension, diabetes mellitus, and coronary artery disease are common antecedents.
- Neurohormonal activation, including sympathetic nervous and renin-angiotensin-aldosterone system activation, and inflammation are common pathogenetic mechanisms that contribute to the progression of heart failure.
- The diagnosis of heart failure is made after careful history and physical examination and may require additional diagnostic tests, including echocardiography and laboratory tests.
- Pharmacotherapeutics for heart failure target neurohormonal activation and the consequences thereof and effective engagement in self-care is also important in overall heart failure management.

INTRODUCTION

Heart failure (HF) is a worldwide epidemic.[1] The common end point of highly prevalent cardiovascular disorders like hypertension[2] and coronary artery disease,[3] HF currently affects more than 5 million Americans.[4] HF is the most common reason for hospitalization and rehospitalization among older adults,[5] and is the fastest growing cardiovascular disorder in the United States.[6] There are more than 1 million hospital admissions[7] and 3 million emergent visits for HF in the United States annually,[8] which account for 20% of Medicare's hospital payments.[9] With an increase in prevalence, the already large direct cost of HF is expected to triple in the next 20 years.[10] Only 50% of patients live for 5 years after the diagnosis of HF,[11] and those living with HF experience significant symptom burden, functional limitations,[12] and decreased health-related quality of life (HRQOL).[13] Thus, despite decades of advances in therapeutics and knowledge of HF pathogenesis,[14] there are considerable opportunities to

Disclosure: The authors have nothing to disclose.
School of Nursing & Knight Cardiovascular Institute, Oregon Health & Science University, Mail Code: SN-2N, 3455 Southwest US Veterans Hospital Road, Portland, OR 97239-2941, USA
* Corresponding author.
E-mail address: leechri@ohsu.edu

reduce both the national and personal burdens of HF.[15] This article reviews the definition, common causal and pathogenic mechanisms, diagnosis, and treatment of chronic HF.

HEART FAILURE DEFINED

HF is a complex and multisystem clinical syndrome resulting from impaired ventricular contractility and/or relaxation.[16] HF generally results from cardiac muscle dysfunction and is characterized by ventricular dilatation and/or hypertrophy, venous congestion, and inadequate oxygen delivery.[17] There are several subclassifications of HF based on left ventricular ejection fraction (LVEF),[16] which are presented in **Table 1**. The severity of HF is often classified using the New York Heart Association (NYHA) functional classification, which stratifies activity limitations and symptom provocation. Specifically, HF and the treatment thereof can result in no ordinary physical activity limitations or symptoms (NYHA class I); slight limitations to physical activity, no symptoms at rest, but HF symptoms with ordinary physical activity (NYHA class II); comfort at rest with marked limitations to physical activity and HF symptoms with less than ordinary activity (NYHA class III); or the inability to engage in any physical activity without HF symptoms or HF symptoms at rest (NYHA class IV).[18] The American College of Cardiology (ACC) and American Heart Association (AHA) also have a rubric for staging the progressive nature of HF: high risk for the development of HF without structural abnormalities or symptoms (stage A), structural abnormalities without prior or current HF signs or symptoms (stage B), structural abnormalities with prior or current HF symptoms (stage C), and refractory HF requiring advanced therapies (stage D).[19] Collectively, these definitions are used to grade the current impact of HF and its treatment on patients' physical activity as well as to comment on the stage of HF progression.

COMMON CAUSAL PATHWAYS TO HEART FAILURE

Hypertension is a common antecedent to HF.[20,21] In response to increased pressure load and reduced compliance, the left ventricle is altered in both structure and form to accommodate hypertension[22] in HF in general and in HF with preserved ejection fraction in particular.[23] Diabetes mellitus is also a common antecedent to HF.[24,25] Via metabolic disturbances, fibrosis, small vessel accumulation of advanced glycation end products, impaired calcium homeostasis, and insulin resistance, diabetes mellitus is associated with both systolic and diastolic ventricular dysfunction.[26] Coronary artery disease is another common antecedent to HF, because it often results in the loss of functioning cardiomyocytes in addition to ventricular dilatation and fibrosis.[27] There are numerous other causes of HF, including multiple cardiomyopathies (eg,

Table 1
Subclassifications of HF based on ejection fraction

LVEF (%)	Classification	Related Terms
≤40	HFrEF	Systolic heart failure
41–49	Borderline HFpEF, or previous HFrEF that has improved to HFpEF	—
≥50	HFpEF or previous HFrEF that has improved to HFpEF	Diastolic heart failure

Abbreviations: HFpEF, heart failure with preserved ejection fraction; HFrEF, heart failure with reduced ejection fraction.

ischemic, nonischemic, familial, and toxic), valve disease, thyroid disease, and several inflammatory processes that are described in detail elsewhere.[16] In addition, many cases of HF are categorized as idiopathic because of the absence of any specific cause.

PREVAILING PATHOPHYSIOLOGIC MECHANISMS OF HEART FAILURE
Neurohormonal Activation

Despite variations in cause, the cycle of HF pathogenesis typically begins with an insult to the myocardium that causes impaired ventricular contractility and/or relaxation (**Fig. 1**). Reduced arterial filling and blood return to the heart are detected by arterial and cardiopulmonary baroreceptors, respectively, and serve as triggers for sympathetic nervous system (SNS) activation that is largely mediated by the action of norepinephrine on cardiac and vascular smooth muscle cells. The initial functional responses of the SNS to decreased pressure and blood return to the heart involve positive chronotropism (increased heart rate), dromotropism (conduction velocity through the atrioventricular node), inotropism (increased ventricular contractile force), and lusitropism (enhanced ventricular relaxation), as well as vasoconstriction to increase cardiac output, blood pressure, and venous return.[28–30]

In response to both increased circulatory level of norepinephrine from SNS activation and decreased blood pressure in the afferent arterioles of the kidneys, the renin-angiotensin-aldosterone system (RAAS) is also activated in response to impaired

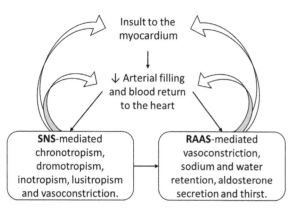

Fig. 1. Cycle of HF pathogenesis. By the actions of the intercellular second messengers of norepinephrine, sympathetic nervous system stimulation of the sinoatrial and atrioventricular node tissue results in higher heart rate (positive chronotropism) and greater conduction velocity (positive dromotropism), respectively. Within cardiomyocytes, the intercellular second messengers of norepinephrine cause greater force of contraction (positive inotropism) and enhanced ventricular relaxation (positive lusitropism). Renin-angiotensin-aldosterone system activation is largely mediated through the intracellular second messengers of angiotensin II on vascular smooth muscle cells (resulting in vasoconstriction), afferent and efferent renal arterioles (resulting in sodium and water retention in the kidney), zona glomerulosa cells of the adrenal glands (resulting in aldosterone secretion), and the median optic nucleus and subfornical organ (resulting in thirst). These initial responses to decreased arterial filling and blood return to the heart are highly functional and help to restore blood pressure and volume. Chronic activation of these and other neurohormonal systems increases myocardial oxygen demand, promotes intracellular calcium toxicity, and causes chamber hypertrophy, fibrosis, and apoptosis, which further impair myocardial function. RAAS, renin-angiotensin-aldosterone system; SNS, sympathetic nervous system.

ventricular contractility and/or relaxation (see **Fig. 1**). As an important regulator of sodium and water balance, RAAS activation results in vasoconstriction, sodium and water retention in the kidney, aldosterone secretion, and increased thirst, which are largely mediated by the actions of angiotensin II on various tissue receptors.[31–33] Collectively, these highly functional responses of RAAS activation cause greater blood volume and higher blood pressure.

Despite initial functional responses, chronic SNS and RAAS activation increase myocardial oxygen demand, promote intracellular calcium toxicity, and give rise to detrimental proliferative remodeling effects such as hypertrophy, fibrosis, and apoptosis.[34–36] Thus, chronic SNS and RAAS activation cause further insult to the myocardium (see **Fig. 1**). The role of SNS and RAAS activation in the pathogenesis of HF remodeling is referred to as the neurohormonal hypothesis[37] and serves as the basis for most evidence-based pharmacologic therapies used in the treatment of HF.

Inflammation

Inflammation also plays a crucial role in the pathophysiology of HF. Thus, the cytokine hypothesis[38] has gained considerable attention in the context of HF. Specifically, several proinflammatory cytokines are expressed in the failing heart that both modulate and contribute to the pathophysiology of HF.[38] Dominant mechanisms of proinflammatory cytokine activity and actions in HF are presented in **Fig. 2**. In brief, shear stress and mechanical overload,[39] mechanical stretch of cardiomyocytes,[40] infection,[41] and tissue ischemia[40] can induce proinflammatory cytokine production in HF. The proinflammatory state is problematic in HF because of the associated adrenergic receptor uncoupling,[39] negative inotropism and lusitropism,[42] nitric oxide synthesis,[39] reactive oxygen species induction,[43] apoptosis, and remodeling.[44] Improving ventricular function and oxygen delivery, reducing the effects of neurohormonal activation such as sodium and water retention and vasoconstriction, limiting

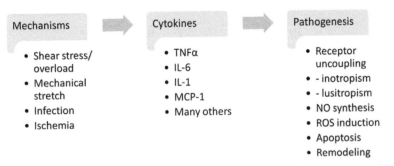

Fig. 2. Role of inflammation in HF. Several proinflammatory cytokines are expressed in the failing heart by shear stress and mechanical overload, which cause endothelial disruption and leukocyte adhesion, mechanical stretch of myocytes, infection as a result of bacterial endotoxin translocation from the gut to the blood during episodes of congestion, and/or by tissue ischemia signaling. Several cytokines have been implicated in uncoupling adrenergic receptors from G proteins; impairing calcium release during systole and removal during diastole, which results in negative inotropism and lusitropism; both calcium dependent and independent nitric oxide synthesis; induction of reactive oxygen species and several other apoptotic mechanisms; and remodeling, including hypertrophy, fibrosis, and expression of noncontractile proteins. IL, interleukin; MCP-1, monocyte chemoattractant protein-1; NO, nitric oxide; ROS, reactive oxygen species; TNFα, tumor necrosis factor alpha.

mechanical overload, and mitigating remodeling of the heart are the main therapeutic targets of both pharmacologic and nonpharmacologic therapies used in the management of HF.

DIAGNOSING HEART FAILURE

The diagnosis of HF can be challenging. Although hallmark symptoms of HF like dyspnea and fatigue often trigger patients to seek medical evaluation, symptoms can be nonspecific and attributed to other conditions or advancing age. Delays in patients' recognition of symptoms and providers' timely diagnosis are impediments to effective HF management. The ACC/AHA,[16] Heart Failure Society of America,[17] and the European Society of Cardiology[45] have all developed detailed guidelines on the diagnosis, evaluation, and treatment of HF.

History and Physical

Each of the evidence-based guidelines stress the importance of a detailed history in the evaluation of HF to identify symptoms, risk factors (including familial conditions like cardiomyopathy that may indicate HF), clues to cause, and both the duration and severity of HF. Common symptoms of HF include dyspnea at rest or with exertion, fatigue and weakness, orthopnea, chest pain/pressure and palpitations, nocturia, and anorexia or nausea. Risk factors such diabetes mellitus, prior myocardial infarct, or a family history of sudden cardiac death in combination with the patient's report of symptoms are indications for further evaluation of HF. Equally important to a detailed history is a comprehensive physical examination.[16,17] Physical examination findings suggestive of HF are presented in **Table 2**, and the commonly used Framingham criteria for the diagnosis of HF are presented in **Table 3**.[46]

Diagnostics

Once HF is suspected, the diagnosis is confirmed with objective measures of cardiac structural defects or dysfunction. Echocardiography is the primary tool to examine the cardiac chamber volumes and structures within the heart.[16,17] An echocardiogram provides information on ventricular volumes, ejection fraction, and systolic and diastolic function, and allows visualization of the valves and wall thickness. Obtaining a

---

Table 2
Clinical examinations findings suggestive of HF

Examination Finding	Clinical Relevance in HF
Jugular venous distention	Volume overload
Hepatojugular reflex	Volume overload
S3 heart sound	Volume overload
Tachycardia	SNS activation
Weak or thready pulse	Decreased cardiac output
Rales/acute pulmonary edema	Volume overload
Dependent edema	Volume overload
Laterally displaced apical pulse	Cardiomegaly/left ventricular dilatation
Murmur	Valvular cause/involvement
Cool extremities	Decreased cardiac output
Decreased capillary refill	Decreased cardiac output

Table 3
Framingham criteria for the diagnosis of HF

Major Criteria	Minor Criteria
Paroxysmal nocturnal dyspnea	Nocturnal cough
Weight loss of 4.5 kg in 5 d in response to treatment	Dyspnea on exertion
Neck vein distention	A decrease in vital capacity by one-third maximum
Rales	Pleural effusion
Acute pulmonary edema	Tachycardia (rate $\geq$120 beats per min)
Hepatojugular reflux	Bilateral ankle edema
S3 gallop	—
Central venous pressure >16 cm H_2O	—
Circulation time of 25 s	—
Radiographic cardiomegaly	—
Pulmonary edema, visceral congestion, or cardiomegaly at autopsy	—

Note: 2 major criteria or 1 major and 2 minor criteria confer the diagnosis of HF.
From Ho KK, Pinsky JL, Kannel WB, et al. The epidemiology of heart failure: the Framingham Study. J Am Coll Cardiol 1993;22(4 Suppl A):7A; with permission.

chest radiograph is important to assess the size of the heart relative to the thoracic cavity, to provide evidence of pulmonary congestion, and to rule out gross pulmonary causes of symptoms. An electrocardiogram is needed to evaluate rhythm and/or conduction abnormalities that may contribute to symptoms or development of HF and/or warrant additional medications or device therapy.[16,17] Results of these diagnostic tests provide additional objective data that can complement physical examination findings to support the diagnosis of HF.

In cases in which clinical uncertainty exists or echocardiography is not readily available, measurement of B-type natriuretic peptide (BNP) or the amino terminal of BNP (NT-proBNP) can assist with decision making regarding the diagnosis of HF in combination with physical examination findings.[16,17] There are several specific cutoff values for BNP and NT-proBNP that are sensitive and specific enough to help confirm the diagnosis of HF with several caveats. For example, there are several factors that alter BNP and NT-proBNP values, including the degree of myocardial stress, but also kidney failure, pulmonary hypertension, age, gender, and body mass index.[16,17] Hence, levels of BNP and NT-proBNP need to be interpreted with caution. Several other laboratory tests may be needed at the time of diagnosis to rule out additional causes of symptoms, assess the physiologic impact of HF, and to plan appropriate treatment. A complete blood count; urinalysis; serum electrolyte, blood urea nitrogen, serum creatinine, and glucose levels; fasting lipid profile; liver function test; and thyroid-stimulating hormone level are common laboratory tests that can establish a baseline for the initiation of optimal therapy and provide a comparison to evaluate effectiveness of treatment.

Importance of Symptoms in Heart Failure

Symptoms are of paramount importance in HF because changes in symptoms are the primary reason why patients seek urgent therapy.[47–51] Although dyspnea and fatigue are hallmark symptoms of HF, the multiple symptoms experienced by adults with HF are intricately related,[52–55] and several physical and/or affective symptom clusters have been identified and associated with clinical event risk.[52,56,57] Symptoms are also key determinants of HF self-care behaviors, because physical symptoms motivate patients with HF to engage in more effective symptom management strategies,[58–60] and psychological symptoms like depression are significant barriers to self-care.[61–63] In addition, symptoms are also the principal drivers of HRQOL in HF.[64,65] Thus, symptoms are not only important to the diagnosis but also provide important information about clinical and patient-oriented outcomes in HF.

HEART FAILURE MANAGEMENT STRATEGIES

The foundation of HF management involves the initiation of beta-adrenergic blockers and angiotensin-converting enzyme inhibitors to reduce cardiac oxygen demand, improve ventricular function, reduce afterload, mitigate sodium and water retention, and delay ventricular remodeling. The major classes of pharmacologic agents used in the management of HF, including examples and rationales for use, are presented in **Table 4**. Nonpharmacologic strategies can be used to further manage volume overload, improve symptoms, and optimize functional capacity and quality of life. Commonly used strategies include sodium-restricted diets (2–3 g daily) and fluid restriction of 2 L or less daily in those experiencing hyponatremia or fluid retention that is difficult to control.[17] Additional nonpharmacologic therapies that have been shown to improve outcomes are regular exercise, smoking cessation counseling, and treatment of other medical problems, such as sleep apnea and depression.[17]

Table 4
Major drugs used in the management of HF

Class	Examples	Rationale
Beta-adrenergic blockers	Bisoprolol Metoprolol Carvedilol	Partially block SNS Reduce cardiac oxygen demand Improve ventricular function Reduce mortality Decrease hospitalizations
ACE inhibitors	Enalapril Captopril Lisinopril	Partially block RAAS Reduce blood pressure/reduce afterload Reduce sodium and water retention Delay remodeling
Angiotensin receptor blockers	Valsartan Candesartan Losartan	Partially block RAAS Reduce blood pressure/reduce afterload Reduce sodium and water retention Useful for ACE intolerance
Aldosterone receptor antagonists	Spironolactone Eplerenone	Reduce sodium and water retention
Diuretics	Furosemide Bumetanide Torsemide	Reduce congestion Improve symptoms of dyspnea and edema
Digoxin	Digoxin	Controls the ventricular response to atrial fibrillation Improves symptoms Enhances contractility
Vasodilators	Hydralazine Isosorbide dinitrate	Reduce blood pressure/reduce afterload

Abbreviation: ACE, angiotensin-converting enzyme.

When symptoms of HF become refractory to optimal medical therapy, management of advanced HF through referral to a specialist in advanced HF can be beneficial.[66] Definitions of advanced HF and major management options thereof are presented in **Table 5**.

Heart Failure Self-care

Even when patients with HF are treated by expert clinicians and prescribed evidence-based therapies, they are responsible for most of their own care.[67] Self-care maintenance (ie, daily adherence behaviors) is an essential element of the management of HF.[59,62,68] Another necessary and difficult component of self-care is the ability to recognize, evaluate, and subsequently manage symptoms when they occur (ie, self-care management).[67] Better HF self-care is associated with better health status,[69] lower clinical event risk,[70] reduced hemodynamic congestion,[71] less myocardial stress and systemic inflammation,[58] and better quality of life.[72] The inability to recognize HF symptoms has also been associated with delays in seeking treatment of HF.[73,74] Importantly, self-care is highly variable and generally poor among adults with HF.[75–77] Hence, there is an important role for clinicians in promoting effective self-care to allow patients to have greater influence on their own health. Although HF-specific caregiving is associated with poor physical and mental health,[78–81] health care providers often both involve and rely on spouses or adult children to help patients monitor, appraise, and manage HF symptoms. In addition, patient-caregiver dyads work together differently to help manage HF,[82–84] and HF in couples who take a collaborative approach to self-care likely has better outcomes.[85–88] Despite extensive research in this area, the best methods for optimizing self-care and caregiver engagement in the management of HF remain unknown.

Note that, despite optimal medical care and self-management, HF is a progressive disorder that can be delayed but infrequently stopped. Thus, therapeutic strategies often have the goal of prolonging life but at the same time are intended to optimize quality of life. Patients and their families vary in preferences for potential trade-offs for duration and quality of life; thus, patients and families should be an integral part of shared decision making when it comes to HF management strategies.

Table 5
Advanced HF definitions and therapeutic options

Common Defining Criteria	Potential Therapeutic Options
>2 hospitalizations for HF in the past year Severe symptoms (NYHA class III or IV) Progressive deterioration of renal function; increase in blood urea nitrogen and creatinine levels Progressive decline in serum sodium level Escalation of diuretics to maintain volume Severe cardiac dysfunction: • Left ventricular ejection fraction <30% • High filling pressures (wedge pressure >16 mm Hg and/or right atrial pressure >12 mm Hg) • Systolic blood pressure <90 mm Hg Functional decline: peak Vo_2 <12–14 mL/kg/min, or 6-min walk test <300 m Frequent cardioverter defibrillator shocks Cardiac cachexia (unintentional weight loss)	• Cardiac resynchronization therapy • Heart transplantation for patients who are eligible • Mechanical circulatory support for patient who meet selection criteria • Long-term inotrope administration • Palliative/end-of-life care

Abbreviation: Vo_2, peak oxygen uptake.

SUMMARY

The common end point of many cardiovascular disorders, HF is a complex syndrome that results from impaired ventricular contractility or relaxation and is a major cause of morbidity and mortality in industrialized nations. The body's functional responses to impaired blood flow and pressure, including SNS and RAAS activation, contribute significantly to the pathogenesis of HF and are the main targets for pharmacotherapy. Prescription of evidence-based therapies and effective engagement of patients and their caregivers are essential elements of HF management. This article reviews the definition, common causal and pathogenic mechanisms, diagnosis, and treatment of chronic HF. Clinicians who are engaged in the management of HF should seek out additional and detailed sources of information, many of which are cited herein, in order to provide contemporary and evidence-based care.

REFERENCES

1. Najafi F, Jamrozik K, Dobson AJ. Understanding the 'epidemic of heart failure': a systematic review of trends in determinants of heart failure. Eur J Heart Fail 2009; 11(5):472–9.
2. Ong KL, Cheung BM, Man YB, et al. Prevalence, awareness, treatment, and control of hypertension among United States adults 1999-2004. Hypertension 2007; 49(1):69–75.
3. Ford ES, Ajani UA, Croft JB, et al. Explaining the decrease in U.S. deaths from coronary disease, 1980-2000. N Engl J Med 2007;356(23):2388–98.
4. Go AS, Mozaffarian D, Roger VL, et al. Heart disease and stroke statistics–2013 update: a report from the American Heart Association. Circulation 2013;127(1): e6–245.
5. Jencks SF, Williams MV, Coleman EA. Rehospitalizations among patients in the Medicare fee-for-service program. N Engl J Med 2009;360(14):1418.
6. Heidenreich PA, Trogdon JG, Khavjou OA, et al. Forecasting the future of cardiovascular disease in the United States: a policy statement from the American Heart Association. Circulation 2011;123(8):933–44.
7. Koelling TM, Chen RS, Lubwama RN, et al. The expanding national burden of heart failure in the United States: the influence of heart failure in women. Am Heart J 2004;147(1):74–8.
8. Burt CW, Schappert SM. Ambulatory care visits to physician offices, hospital outpatient departments, and emergency departments: United States, 1999–2000. Vital Health Stat 13 2004;(157):1–70.
9. Hernandez AF, Greiner MA, Fonarow GC, et al. Relationship between early physician follow-up and 30-day readmission among Medicare beneficiaries hospitalized for heart failure. JAMA 2010;303(17):1716–22.
10. Heidenreich PA, Albert NM, Allen LA, et al. Forecasting the impact of heart failure in the United States: a policy statement from the American Heart Association. Circ Heart Fail 2013;6(3):606–19.
11. Roger VL, Weston SA, Redfield MM, et al. Trends in heart failure incidence and survival in a community-based population. JAMA 2004;292(3):344–50.
12. Moser DK, Doering LV, Chung ML. Vulnerabilities of patients recovering from an exacerbation of chronic heart failure. Am Heart J 2005;150(5):984.
13. Westlake C, Dracup K, Fonarow G, et al. Depression in patients with heart failure. J Card Fail 2005;11(1):30–5.
14. Kosiborod M, Lichtman JH, Heidenreich PA, et al. National trends in outcomes among elderly patients with heart failure. Am J Med 2006;119(7):616.e1–7.

15. Bradley EH, Curry L, Horwitz LI, et al. Contemporary evidence about hospital strategies for reducing 30-day readmissions: a national study. J Am Coll Cardiol 2012;60(7):607–14.
16. Yancy CW, Jessup M, Bozkurt B, et al. 2013 ACCF/AHA guideline for the management of heart failure: a report of the American College of Cardiology Foundation/American Heart Association Task Force on practice guidelines. Circulation 2013;128(16):e240–327.
17. Lindenfeld J, Albert NM, Boehmer JP, et al. HFSA 2010 comprehensive heart failure practice guideline. J Card Fail 2010;16(6):e1–194.
18. Fisher JD. New York Heart Association classification. Arch Intern Med 1972; 129(5):836.
19. Hunt SA, Abraham WT, Chin MH, et al. 2009 focused update incorporated into the ACC/AHA 2005 guidelines for the diagnosis and management of heart failure in adults: a report of the American College of Cardiology Foundation/American Heart Association Task Force on Practice Guidelines: developed in collaboration with the International Society for Heart and Lung Transplantation. Circulation 2009;119(14):e391–479.
20. Levy D, Larson MG, Vasan RS, et al. The progression from hypertension to congestive heart failure. JAMA 1996;275(20):1557–62.
21. Lloyd-Jones DM, Larson MG, Leip EP, et al. Lifetime risk for developing congestive heart failure: the Framingham Heart Study. Circulation 2002;106(24):3068–72.
22. Mayet J, Hughes A. Cardiac and vascular pathophysiology in hypertension. Heart 2003;89(9):1104–9.
23. Owan TE, Hodge DO, Herges RM, et al. Trends in prevalence and outcome of heart failure with preserved ejection fraction. N Engl J Med 2006;355(3):251–9.
24. He J, Ogden LG, Bazzano LA, et al. Risk factors for congestive heart failure in US men and women: NHANES I epidemiologic follow-up study. Arch Intern Med 2001;161(7):996–1002.
25. Kenchaiah S, Evans JC, Levy D, et al. Obesity and the risk of heart failure. N Engl J Med 2002;347(5):305–13.
26. Kasznicki J, Drzewoski J. Heart failure in the diabetic population - pathophysiology, diagnosis and management. Arch Med Sci 2014;10(3):546–56.
27. Gheorghiade M, Sopko G, De Luca L, et al. Navigating the crossroads of coronary artery disease and heart failure. Circulation 2006;114(11):1202–13.
28. Schrier RW, Abraham WT. Hormones and hemodynamics in heart failure. N Engl J Med 1999;341(8):577–85.
29. Kjaer A, Hesse B. Heart failure and neuroendocrine activation: diagnostic, prognostic and therapeutic perspectives. Clin Physiol 2001;21(6):661–72.
30. Yamanaka T, Onishi K, Tanabe M, et al. Force- and relaxation-frequency relations in patients with diastolic heart failure. Am Heart J 2006;152(5):966.e1–7.
31. Ferrario CM, Strawn WB. Role of the renin-angiotensin-aldosterone system and proinflammatory mediators in cardiovascular disease. Am J Cardiol 2006;98(1):121–8.
32. Carey RM, Siragy HM. Newly recognized components of the renin-angiotensin system: potential roles in cardiovascular and renal regulation. Endocr Rev 2003;24(3):261–71.
33. McKinley MJ, Cairns MJ, Denton DA, et al. Physiological and pathophysiological influences on thirst. Physiol Behav 2004;81(5):795–803.
34. Katz AM. Heart failure: a hemodynamic disorder complicated by maladaptive proliferative responses. J Cell Mol Med 2003;7(1):1–10.
35. Struthers AD. Pathophysiology of heart failure following myocardial infarction. Heart 2005;91(Suppl 2):ii14–6 [discussion: ii31, ii43–8].

36. Henrion D, Kubis N, Levy BI. Physiological and pathophysiological functions of the AT(2) subtype receptor of angiotensin II: from large arteries to the microcirculation. Hypertension 2001;38(5):1150–7.
37. Packer M. The neurohormonal hypothesis: a theory to explain the mechanism of disease progression in heart failure. J Am Coll Cardiol 1992;20(1):248–54.
38. Seta Y, Shan K, Bozkurt B, et al. Basic mechanisms in heart failure: the cytokine hypothesis. J Card Fail 1996;2(3):243–9.
39. Aukrust P, Gullestad L, Ueland T, et al. Inflammatory and anti-inflammatory cytokines in chronic heart failure: potential therapeutic implications. Ann Med 2005; 37(2):74–85.
40. Nian M, Lee P, Khaper N, et al. Inflammatory cytokines and postmyocardial infarction remodeling. Circ Res 2004;94(12):1543–53.
41. Peschel T, Schonauer M, Thiele H, et al. Invasive assessment of bacterial endotoxin and inflammatory cytokines in patients with acute heart failure. Eur J Heart Fail 2003;5(5):609–14.
42. Hedayat M, Mahmoudi MJ, Rose NR, et al. Proinflammatory cytokines in heart failure: double-edged swords. Heart Fail Rev 2010;15(6):543–62.
43. Lopez Farre A, Casado S. Heart failure, redox alterations, and endothelial dysfunction. Hypertension 2001;38(6):1400–5.
44. Mann DL. Inflammatory mediators and the failing heart: past, present, and the foreseeable future. Circ Res 2002;91(11):988–98.
45. McMurray JJ, Adamopoulos S, Anker SD, et al. ESC guidelines for the diagnosis and treatment of acute and chronic heart failure 2012: the Task Force for the Diagnosis and Treatment of Acute and Chronic Heart Failure 2012 of the European Society of Cardiology. Developed in collaboration with the Heart Failure Association (HFA) of the ESC. Eur J Heart Fail 2012;14(8):803–69.
46. Ho KK, Pinsky JL, Kannel WB, et al. The epidemiology of heart failure: the Framingham Study. J Am Coll Cardiol 1993;22(4 Suppl A):6A–13A.
47. Adams KF Jr, Fonarow GC, Emerman CL, et al. Characteristics and outcomes of patients hospitalized for heart failure in the United States: rationale, design, and preliminary observations from the first 100,000 cases in the Acute Decompensated Heart Failure National Registry (ADHERE). Am Heart J 2005;149(2):209–16.
48. Gheorghiade M, Zannad F, Sopko G, et al. Acute heart failure syndromes: current state and framework for future research. Circulation 2005;112(25):3958–68.
49. Felker GM, Leimberger JD, Califf RM, et al. Risk stratification after hospitalization for decompensated heart failure. J Card Fail 2004;10(6):460–6.
50. De Luca L, Fonarow GC, Adams KF Jr, et al. Acute heart failure syndromes: clinical scenarios and pathophysiologic targets for therapy. Heart Fail Rev 2007; 12(2):97–104.
51. Goldberg RJ, Spencer FA, Szklo-Coxe M, et al. Symptom presentation in patients hospitalized with acute heart failure. Clin Cardiol 2010;33(6):E73–80.
52. Lee CS, Gelow JM, Denfeld QE, et al. Physical and psychological symptom profiling and event-free survival in adults with moderate to advanced heart failure. J Cardiovasc Nurs 2014;29(4):315–23.
53. Rector TS. A conceptual model of quality of life in relation to heart failure. J Card Fail 2005;11(3):173–6.
54. Song EK, Moser DK, Lennie TA. Relationship of depressive symptoms to the impact of physical symptoms on functional status in women with heart failure. Am J Crit Care 2009;18(4):348–56.
55. De Jong MJ, Chung ML, Wu JR, et al. Linkages between anxiety and outcomes in heart failure. Heart Lung 2011;40(5):393–404.

56. Lee KS, Song EK, Lennie TA, et al. Symptom clusters in men and women with heart failure and their impact on cardiac event-free survival. J Cardiovasc Nurs 2010;25(4):263–72.

57. Song EK, Moser DK, Rayens MK, et al. Symptom clusters predict event-free survival in patients with heart failure. J Cardiovasc Nurs 2010;25(4):284–91.

58. Lee CS, Moser DK, Lennie TA, et al. Biomarkers of myocardial stress and systemic inflammation in patients who engage in heart failure self-care management. J Cardiovasc Nurs 2011;26(4):321–8.

59. Riegel B, Lee CS, Albert N, et al. From novice to expert: confidence and activity status determine heart failure self-care performance. Nurs Res 2011;60(2):132–8.

60. Lee CS, Gelow JM, Mudd JO, et al. Profiles of self-care management versus consulting behaviors in adults with heart failure. Eur J Cardiovasc Nurs 2015; 14(1):63–72.

61. Pelle AJ, Schiffer AA, Smith OR, et al. Inadequate consultation behavior modulates the relationship between type D personality and impaired health status in chronic heart failure. Int J Cardiol 2010;142(1):65–71.

62. Moser DK, Dickson V, Jaarsma T, et al. Role of self-care in the patient with heart failure. Curr Cardiol Rep 2012;14(3):265–75.

63. Oosterom-Calo R, van Ballegooijen AJ, Terwee CB, et al. Determinants of heart failure self-care: a systematic literature review. Heart Fail Rev 2012;17(3):367–85.

64. Bekelman DB, Havranek EP, Becker DM, et al. Symptoms, depression, and quality of life in patients with heart failure. J Card Fail 2007;13(8):643–8.

65. Zambroski CH, Moser DK, Bhat G, et al. Impact of symptom prevalence and symptom burden on quality of life in patients with heart failure. Eur J Cardiovasc Nurs 2005;4(3):198–206.

66. Fang JC, Ewald GA, Allen LA, et al. Advanced (stage D) heart failure: a statement from the Heart Failure Society of America Guidelines Committee. J Card Fail 2015;21(6):519–34.

67. Riegel B, Moser DK, Anker SD, et al. State of the science: promoting self-care in persons with heart failure: a scientific statement from the American Heart Association. Circulation 2009;120(12):1141–63.

68. Riegel B, Dickson VV. A situation-specific theory of heart failure self-care. J Cardiovasc Nurs 2008;23:190–6.

69. Lee CS, Suwanno J, Riegel B. The relationship between self-care and health status domains in Thai patients with heart failure. Eur J Cardiovasc Nurs 2009;8(4):259–66.

70. Lee CS, Moser DK, Lennie TA, et al. Event-free survival in adults with heart failure who engage in self-care management. Heart Lung 2011;40(1):12–20.

71. Rathman LD, Lee CS, Sarkar S, et al. A critical link between heart failure self-care and intrathoracic impedance. J Cardiovasc Nurs 2011;26(4):E20–6.

72. Lee CS, Mudd JO, Hiatt SO, et al. Trajectories of heart failure self-care management and changes in quality of life. Eur J Cardiovasc Nurs 2014. [Epub ahead of print].

73. Jurgens CY. Somatic awareness, uncertainty, and delay in care-seeking in acute heart failure. Res Nurs Health 2006;29(2):74–86.

74. Gravely-Witte S, Jurgens CY, Tamim H, et al. Length of delay in seeking medical care by patients with heart failure symptoms and the role of symptom-related factors: a narrative review. Eur J Heart Fail 2010;12(10):1122–9.

75. Webel AR, Frazier SK, Lennie T, et al. Daily variability in dyspnea, edema and body weight in heart failure patients. Eur J Cardiovasc Nurs 2007;6(1):60–5.

76. Moser DK, Frazier SK, Worrall-Carter L, et al. Symptom variability, not severity, predicts rehospitalization and mortality in patients with heart failure. Eur J Cardiovasc Nurs 2011;10(2):124–9.

77. Riegel B, Lee CS, Dickson VV. Self care in patients with chronic heart failure. Nat Rev Cardiol 2011;8(11):644–54.
78. Pressler SJ, Gradus-Pizlo I, Chubinski SD, et al. Family caregiver outcomes in heart failure. Am J Crit Care 2009;18(2):149–59.
79. Bakas T, Pressler SJ, Johnson EA, et al. Family caregiving in heart failure. Nurs Res 2006;55(3):180–8.
80. Chung ML, Pressler SJ, Dunbar SB, et al. Predictors of depressive symptoms in caregivers of patients with heart failure. J Cardiovasc Nurs 2010;25(5):411–9.
81. Kang X, Li Z, Nolan MT. Informal caregivers' experiences of caring for patients with chronic heart failure: systematic review and metasynthesis of qualitative studies. J Cardiovasc Nurs 2011;26(5):386–94.
82. Lee CS, Vellone E, Lyons KS, et al. Patterns and predictors of patient and caregiver engagement in heart failure care: a multi-level dyadic study. Int J Nurs Stud 2015;52(2):588–97.
83. Lyons KS, Vellone E, Lee CS, et al. A dyadic approach to managing heart failure with confidence. J Cardiovasc Nurs 2015;30(4 Suppl 1):S64–71.
84. Buck HG, Kitko L, Hupcey JE. Dyadic heart failure care types: qualitative evidence for a novel typology. J Cardiovasc Nurs 2013;28(6):E37–46.
85. Quinn C, Dunbar SB, Higgins M. Heart failure symptom assessment and management: can caregivers serve as proxy? J Cardiovasc Nurs 2010;25:142–8.
86. Retrum JH, Nowels CT, Bekelman DB. Patient and caregiver congruence: the importance of dyads in heart failure care. J Cardiovasc Nurs 2013;28:129–36.
87. Sebern M, Riegel B. Contributions of supportive relationships to heart failure self-care. Eur J Cardiovasc Nurs 2009;8:97–104.
88. Rohrbaugh MJ, Mehl MR, Shoham V, et al. Prognostic significance of spouse we talk in couples coping with heart failure. J Consult Clin Psychol 2008;76:781–9.

Heart Failure and Atrial Fibrillation

Brenda McCulloch, RN, MSN

KEYWORDS

- Atrial fibrillation • Thromboembolism • Rate control • Rhythm control
- Cardioversion • Ablation

KEY POINTS

- Atrial fibrillation is common in patients with heart failure.
- Rate control or rhythm control are 2 important strategies to consider when managing patients with heart failure who are in atrial fibrillation.
- Some patients with heart failure and atrial fibrillation benefit from cardioversion, device therapy with pacemakers or implantable cardioverter defibrillators, catheter, or surgical-based ablation.

INTRODUCTION

Heart failure (HF) and atrial fibrillation (AF) are 2 commonly seen cardiovascular disorders that share multiple risk factors and continue to increase in the United States as well as worldwide. Each increase morbidity and mortality in patients, and when seen together, the impact can be additive because of the complex interaction between the 2 conditions.[1–3]

The burden of AF and HF is projected to surge due to our aging population and increased survival from other cardiovascular disease, especially coronary artery disease. Heart disease continues to be the predominant cause of death in both men and women in the United States. Nearly 6 million Americans suffer from HF and half of those newly diagnosed with HF will die within 5 years.[4] As of 2010, between 2.7 and 6.1 million people in the United States had AF and it is anticipated to be as high as 12 million by 2050 because of its steadily increasing rate.[5]

THE HEART FAILURE–ATRIAL FIBRILLATION CONNECTION

HF and AF cause patients to have uncomfortable and potentially distressing symptoms, increase the risk of stroke, decrease quality of life and reduce longevity, while

The author has no financial or commercial conflicts of interests and has received no funding for this project.
Sutter Medical Center, Sacramento, 2801 L Street, Sacramento, CA 95816, USA
E-mail address: mccullb@sutterhealth.org

Crit Care Nurs Clin N Am 27 (2015) 427–438
http://dx.doi.org/10.1016/j.cnc.2015.07.003
0899-5885/15/$ – see front matter
ccnursing.theclinics.com

increasing health care costs The association between AF and HF has been appreciated for decades, and it is well known that the presence of HF increases the risk of AF, whereas the presence of AF increases the risk of HF.[6,7] This has been described as a vicious cycle. More than 70% of patients with AF have underlying heart disease.[8] The prevalence of AF in those with HF ranges from 4% to 40% as the degree of HF worsens.[1] AF is defined by the duration of episodes of the arrhythmia. See **Table 1** for details about AF classifications.[9]

Although there are many shared risk factors between HF and AF, the pathophysiological relationship between AF and HF is not completely understood. Common risk factors of HF and AF include advanced age, hypertension, diabetes mellitus, coronary artery disease, and valvular heart disease. Additional risk factors for AF have been identified and can be seen in **Box 1**. Goals of therapy include management of symptoms and prevention of thromboembolism. Correction of potential underlying causes is needed as well as optimization of HF treatment.[10,11] Patients with HF with either systolic or diastolic dysfunction are at risk. Systolic HF is associated with a significantly increased risk of AF and is a strong predictor for the development of AF.[12] AF occurs when structural and/or electrophysiological abnormalities alter atrial tissue to promote abnormal impulse formation and/or propagation.[9]

AF is an uncoordinated supraventricular arrhythmia in which there is loss of atrial synchrony. This results in the loss of atrial contribution to the cardiac output, commonly referred to as loss of atrial kick.[13] Atrial contraction contributes 20% to 25% of left ventricular stroke volume.[8,12] This reduction in stroke volume leads to reduced cardiac output and lowered exercise tolerance. AF may cause valvular regurgitation, which causes reduction in forward blood flow. Rapid ventricular rates during periods of uncontrolled AF lead to inadequate ventricle filling time and decrease in stroke volume. An irregular ventricular response, in itself and independent of heart rate, causes a drop in cardiac output, increase in pulmonary wedge pressure, and elevation of right atrial pressure.[12]

The detrimental effects of AF on HF also may be worsened by antiarrhythmic therapy. Some antiarrhythmic drugs have negative inotropic effects, whereas others are considered proarrhythmic, meaning that it worsens existing arrhythmias or causes

Table 1
Classification of atrial fibrillation

AF Type	Duration
Paroxysmal AF	AF that terminates spontaneously or with intervention within 7 d of onset. Episodes may recur with variable frequency.
Persistent AF	Continuous AF that is sustained >7 d.
Long-standing persistent AF	Continuous AF >12 mo in duration.
Permanent AF	The term "permanent AF" is used when the patient and clinician make a joint decision to stop further attempts to restore and/or maintain sinus rhythm.
Nonvalvular AF	AF in the absence of rheumatic mitral stenosis, a mechanical or bioprosthetic heart valve, or mitral valve repair.

Abbreviation: AF, atrial fibrillation.
From January CT, Wann LS, Alpert JS, et al. 2014 AHA/ACC/HRS guideline for the management of patients with atrial fibrillation: executive summary: a report of the American College of Cardiology/American Heart Association Task Force on Practice Guidelines and the Heart Rhythm Society. J Am Coll Cardiol 2014;64:2246–80; with permission.

Box 1
Risk factors for atrial fibrillation

- Many cardiovascular diseases, including cardiomyopathy, cardiothoracic surgery, heart failure, hypertension, myocardial infarction, myocarditis, pericarditis, pulmonary embolism, valvular heart disease
- Alcohol use, binge drinking
- Diabetes mellitus
- Electrocution
- Family history, European ancestry, genetic variants
- Exercise
- Hyperthyroidism
- Increasing age
- Obesity
- Obstructive sleep apnea
- Pneumonia
- Smoking

Data from January CT, Wann LS, Alpert JS, et al. 2014 AHA/ACC/HRS guideline for the management of patients with atrial fibrillation: executive summary: a report of the American College of Cardiology/American Heart Association Task Force on Practice Guidelines and the Heart Rhythm Society. J Am Coll Cardiol 2014;64:2246–80; and Sharma AK, Mansour M, Ruskin JN, et al. Atrial fibrillation and congestive heart failure. The Journal of Innovations in Cardiac Rhythm Management 2011;2:253–62.

---

new arrhythmias.[6] Currently there are only 2 antiarrhythmic agents (amiodarone and dofetilide) that are recommended in current guidelines for patients with HF and AF.[9]

When treating patients with HF and AF, key strategies include thromboembolism to prevent stroke, control of heart rate to prevent further ventricular damage, and restore sinus rhythm for patients who would most benefit.

ANTICOAGULATION

There is a significant risk of thromboembolism in AF. In nonvalvular AF, the risk of stroke is increased 5 times, whereas AF in the setting of mitral stenosis increases the risk of stroke 20 times. Additionally, patients have a greater risk of recurrent stroke, more severe disability, and higher death rate. Anticoagulation therapy is indicated to reduce clot formation in the left atrium (LA) or left atrial appendage (LAA). The CHA_2DS_2-VASc tool is recommended for use when assessing stroke risk in patients with nonvalvular AF.[9] In this tool, points are assigned to various risk factors. Risk factors included in the tool can be seen in **Table 2**. For the patient with a score of 0, generally no anticoagulation is indicated. For patients with a score of 1, anticoagulation may be indicated. For patients with a score of 2 or more, anticoagulation is indicated. All anticoagulant agents increase the risk of bleeding and hemorrhage. Anticoagulation medications are detailed in **Table 3**.

Aspirin alone is not recommended for preventing stroke in patients with AF. Warfarin has been used widely for decades,[1,12] yet there are challenges with its use that require provider and physician discussion, including a slow onset of action, narrow

Table 2
CHA$_2$DS$_2$-VASc risk tool

Points		Risk Factors
1	C	Congestive heart failure/left ventricular dysfunction
1	H	Hypertension
2	A2	Age $\geq$ 75 y
1	D	Diabetes mellitus
2	S	Stroke/Transient ischemic attack/Thromboembolism
1	V	Vascular disease, coronary disease, myocardial infarction, peripheral arterial disease, aortic plaque
1	A	Age 65–74
1	S	Sex category – female gender

From January CT, Wann LS, Alpert JS, et al. 2014 AHA/ACC/HRS guideline for the management of patients with atrial fibrillation: executive summary: a report of the American College of Cardiology/American Heart Association Task Force on Practice Guidelines and the Heart Rhythm Society. J Am Coll Cardiol 2014;64:2246–80; with permission.

therapeutic window, interactions with other drugs, effects of alterations in diet, and the requirement for close monitoring with frequent international normalized ratio testing. Additionally, it has been demonstrated that patients may not be within therapeutic range as much as 50% of the time.[9]

Newer options now available for patient with nonvalvular AF include dabigatran, rivaroxaban, or apixaban.[9] These newer oral anticoagulants do not require the need for frequent monitoring. It is anticipated that these agents will partially replace the use of warfarin, but higher cost may be a limiting factor for patients. Current guidelines promote the importance of shared decision-making with the patient, including discussion of cost, patient preference regarding the choice of anticoagulant, and patients and their families need to be well-educated about taking anticoagulants.

RATE CONTROL

Rate control, where the heart rate is controlled but the patient remains in AF, is an important strategy in managing patients to prevent hemodynamic compromise. Medications most commonly used for this include beta blockers, calcium channel blockers, and digoxin, and are detailed in **Table 4**. The goal of rate control is to keep the resting heart rate between 60 and 80 beats per minute or 90 to 115 beats per minute during exercise.[13] Rhythm control, or restoration of sinus rhythm, is beneficial for many patients, especially those who are younger, as it maintains their quality of life, reduces morbidity, and decreases the potential for developing tachycardia-induced cardiomyopathy. Rhythm control has not been found to be superior to rate control.

In patients with acutely decompensated HF and AF, the initial treatment includes intravenous medications to slow the ventricular response, diuretics, and vasodilators. When very rapid control of ventricular rate in AF is required in the hemodynamically compromised patient, electrical cardioversion may be used, although it may increase the risk of a thromboembolic stroke in patients inadequately anticoagulated or for whom AF is of uncertain duration. The administration of beta blockers is beneficial for rate control, once the patient's hemodynamic status is stabilized.

Table 3
Anticoagulation used in atrial fibrillation

Warfarin (Coumadin) Dose dependent on INR	• Preferred for patients with mechanical heart valves; target INR should be based on the type and location of the prosthesis (2.0–3.0 or 2.5–3.5). • For patients with nonvalvular AF, a target INR of 2.0–3.0 is recommended. • Therapeutic INR may not be present for 3–5 d. • INR should be assessed at least weekly during initiation of therapy and at least monthly when INR is in range and stable.
Dabigatran (Pradaxa) 150 mg twice daily; reduce to 75 mg twice daily for patients with decreased creatinine clearance (CrCl) CrCl 15–30 mL/min)	• Direct thrombin inhibitor. • FDA approved for use in nonvalvular AF. • May cause dyspepsia. • Renally excreted. • Dialyzable. • Do not use in patients with AF and a mechanical heart valve. • Not recommended in patients with AF and end-stage CKD or on hemodialysis because of the lack of evidence from clinical trials regarding the balance of risks and benefits.
Rivaroxaban (Xarelto) 20 mg once daily, reduce to 15 mg daily for patients with decreased CrCl (CrCl 15–30 mL/min)	• Factor Xa inhibitor. • FDA approved for use in nonvalvular AF. • Renally excreted. • Not dialyzable. • Not recommended in patients with AF and end-stage CKD or on hemodialysis because of the lack of evidence from clinical trials regarding the balance of risks and benefits.
Apixaban (Eliquis) 5 mg PO twice daily; reduce to 2.5 mg daily if age ≥80 y, body weight ≤60 kg, or serum creatinine ≥1.5 mg/dL	• Factor Xa inhibitor. • FDA approved for use in nonvalvular AF. • Hepatically eliminated. • Not dialyzable.

Abbreviations: AF, atrial fibrillation; CKD, chronic kidney disease; FDA, Food and Drug Administration; INR, international normalized ratio; PO, by mouth.

Data from January CT, Wann LS, Alpert JS, et al. 2014 AHA/ACC/HRS guideline for the management of patients with atrial fibrillation: executive summary: a report of the American College of Cardiology/American Heart Association Task Force on Practice Guidelines and the Heart Rhythm Society. J Am Coll Cardiol 2014;64:2246–80; and Lardizabal JA, Deedwania PC. Atrial fibrillation in heart failure. Med Clin North Am 2012;96:987–1000.

RHYTHM CONTROL

In rhythm control, sinus rhythm is restored using antiarrhythmic drug therapy, cardioversion, or arrhythmia ablation. Key antiarrhythmic medications used in patients with HF include amiodarone and dofetilide.[6] See **Table 5** for information regarding medications used for the pharmacologic conversion of AF to sinus rhythm. Antiarrhythmics have adverse effects, as well as drug–drug interactions. Side effects of antiarrhythmic drugs include torsades de pointes, neuropathy, and thyroid dysfunction, and treatment-related death.[17] A major concern with rhythm control is the risk of ventricular proarrhythmias.[8] **Table 6** describes medications used to maintain sinus rhythm once it is obtained.

Table 4
Medications for rate control

Beta blockers
Atenolol (Tenormin) 25–100 mg PO daily
Bisoprolol (Zebeta) 2.5–10 mg PO daily
Carvedilol (Coreg) 3.125–25 mg PO twice daily
Esmolol (Brevibloc) 500 µg/kg IV bolus over
  1 min, then 50–300 µg/kg/min continuous
  infusion
Metoprolol tartrate (Lopressor) 2.5–5 mg IV
  over 5 min; up to 3 doses
Metoprolol XL (succinate) (Toprol XL)
  50–400 mg PO daily
Nadolol (Corgard) 10–240 mg PO daily
Propranolol (Inderal) 1 mg IV over 1 min,
  up to 3 doses at 2-min intervals
	• Beta blockers are useful for ventricular rate control in AF.
	• Use cautiously in acutely decompensated HF.
	• Monitor for bradycardia, hypotension, AV heart block.

Nondihydropyridine calcium channel blockers
Diltiazem (Cardizem) 120–360 mg PO daily
  or 0.25 mg IV with repeat dosing to a
  maximum of 1.5 mg over 24 h
Verapamil (Calan) 180–480 mg PO daily or
  0.075–0.15 mg/kg IV bolus over 2 min;
  may give an additional 10 mg after 30 min
  if no response, then 0.005 mg/kg/min
  continuous infusion
	• Calcium channel blockers have direct AV nodal effect and are useful for ventricular rate control in AF.
	• Use with caution in HF with depressed EF and acute decompensated HF because of negative inotropic effect.
	• Monitor for hypotension, bradycardia, or AV heart block.

Digoxin 0.125–0.25 mg daily or 0.25 mg IV
  with repeat dosing to a maximum of
  1.5 mg over 24 h
	• Second-line drug. Digoxin combined with beta blockers can be effective.
	• Should not be used in conjunction with dronedarone.
	• Monitor potassium levels.
	• Monitor for signs of toxicity.
	• Adverse effects include AV block, ventricular arrhythmias.

Amiodarone (Coradone, Pacerone) 100–200 mg PO daily or 300 mg IV over 1 h, then 10–50 mg/h over 24 h	• Useful for rate control for patients resistant to beta blockers and digoxin. • Multiple dosing schemes exist for amiodarone.
Avoid: Dronedarone (Multaq)	• Contraindicated in patients with decompensated congestive HF and in patients with advanced HF.

Abbreviations: AF, atrial fibrillation; AV, atrioventricular; HF, heart failure; IV, intravenous; PO, by mouth.
   Data from Refs.[6,9,12,14,15]

CARDIOVERSION

Cardioversion with direct-current energy synchronized to the R-wave is commonly performed in patients with AF to restore normal sinus rhythm. A defibrillator providing a biphasic waveform shock is more effective than a monophasic waveform. The initial use of a higher-energy shock (150–200 J) is more effective and may minimize the number of shocks required as well as the duration of sedation. An anterior-posterior paddle/pad placement is often preferred. The overall success rate of cardioversion in AF is greater than 90%, but that decreases as duration of the AF increases.[16]

Table 5
Medications for pharmacologic conversion of AF

Amiodarone (Cordarone, Pacerone) 600–800 mg PO daily in divided doses to a total load of up to 10 g, then 200 mg daily for maintenance Or 150 mg IV over 10 min, then 1 mg/min for 6 h, then 0.5 mg/min for 18 h or change to oral dosing	• Class III antiarrhythmic. • Potential adverse effects include phlebitis, hypotension, bradycardia, QT prolongation, torsade de pointe (rare), GI upset, constipation, increased INR. • Risk of pulmonary, hepatic, and thyroid toxicity.
Dofetilide (Tikosyn) 125–500 mg PO twice daily; dose dependent on creatinine clearance	• Class III antiarrhythmic. • Indicated for the conversion and maintenance of normal sinus rhythm in AF/flutter. • Proarrhythmic; requires hospitalization for careful monitoring during drug initiation due to severe QT interval prolongation and torsades de points in up to 3% of patients. • Negative chronotropic effects. • Contraindicated in congenital long QT syndrome or acquired QT prolongation syndromes, or history of torsade de pointes.
Ibutilide (Corvert) 1 mg IV over 10 min; may repeat once if necessary (if body weight < 60 kg, use 0.01 mg/kg)	• Avoid use in patients with EF < 20%. • Pretreatment with magnesium may prevent torsade de points. • ECG monitoring required for 4 h following administration. • Potential adverse effects include: QT prolongation, torsades de pointes, hypotension.

Abbreviations: AF, atrial fibrillation; ECG, electrocardiogram; EF, ejection fraction; GI, gastrointestinal; INR, international normalized ratio; IV, intravenous; PO, by mouth.
Data from Refs.[11,15,16]

If the patient is hemodynamically unstable due to a rapid ventricular response, intravenous medications or electrical cardioversion may be used to control the heart rate. Electrical cardioversion is preferred in patients with decompensated HF, ongoing myocardial ischemia, or hypotension. However, if the patient is not anticoagulated, there is an increased risk of stroke.

Patients with AF lasting more than 48 hours should be anticoagulated for 3 weeks before planned cardioversion to reduce the risk of stroke. A transesophageal echocardiogram (TEE) may be indicated to exclude the presence of atrial thrombus before the cardioversion. It is more sensitive and specific than the standard transthoracic approach to detect LA thrombi as a potential source of systemic embolism in AF. TEE can also identify features associated with an increased risk of LA thrombus formation, including reduced LAA flow velocity, spontaneous LA contrast, and aortic atheroma.[9]

Cardioversion is typically done in the outpatient/hospital setting using procedural sedation. Before elective cardioversion, the patient should be assessed for digoxin toxicity, hypokalemia, and other electrolyte imbalances. These should be corrected before cardioversion is attempted. Risks of cardioversion include thromboembolism, sedation-related complications, ventricular tachycardia and fibrillation, bradyarrhythmias, skin burn or irritation from electrodes, muscle soreness, and reprogramming or altering implanted cardiac device function.[9,16] If the initial cardioversion is unsuccessful, repeated attempts may be made after adjusting the location of the electrodes, applying pressure over the electrodes, or following administration of an antiarrhythmic medication, such as sotalol, ibutilide, or dofetilide.

Table 6
Maintenance of sinus rhythm in AF

Disopyramide (Norpace) Immediate release: 100–200 mg every 6 h Extended release: 200–400 mg every 12 h	Use with caution in HF, prolonged QT interval, prostatism, glaucoma; avoid other QT prolonging medications.
Quinidine 324–648 mg every 8 h	Prolongs QT interval.
Flecainide (Tambocor) 50–200 mg once every 12 h	• Class IC antiarrhythmic. • Use with caution in HF, SA node/AV node dysfunction, renal or liver disease.
Propafenone (Rythmol) Immediate release: 150–300 mg once every 8 h Extended release: 225–425 mg once every 12 h	• Class IC antiarrhythmic. • Use with caution in HF, SA node/AV node dysfunction, liver disease, asthma.
Amiodarone (Cordarone, Pacerone) 400–600 mg daily in divided doses for 2–4 wk; maintenance typically 100–200 mg daily	• Class III antiarrhythmic • Use with caution in SA node/AV node dysfunction, lung disease, or prolonged QT interval.
Dofetilide (Tikosyn) 125–500 µg once every 12 h	• Class III antiarrhythmic. • Use with caution in renal disease, diuretic therapy, prolonged QT, hypokalemia, hypomagnesemia, avoid other QT prolonging medications.
Sotalol (Betapace) 40–160 mg once every 12 h	• Class III antiarrhythmic. • Use with caution in HF, renal disease, diuretic therapy, prolonged QT, hypokalemia, hypomagnesemia, avoid other QT prolonging medications, SA node/AV node dysfunction, asthma.
Dronedarone (Multaq) should not be used for treatment of AF in patients with NYHA class III and IV HF or patients who have had an episode of decompensated HF in the past 4 wk	Class III antiarrhythmic.

Abbreviations: AF, atrial fibrillation; AV, atrioventricular; HF, heart failure; NYHA, New York Heart Association; SA, sinoatrial.

Data from January CT, Wann LS, Alpert JS, et al. 2014 AHA/ACC/HRS guideline for the management of patients with atrial fibrillation: executive summary: a report of the American College of Cardiology/American Heart Association Task Force on Practice Guidelines and the Heart Rhythm Society. J Am Coll Cardiol 2014;64:2246–80; and Prasun MA. Providing best practice in the management of atrial fibrillation in the United States. J Cardiovasc Nurs 2012;27(5):445–56.

Patients who may not benefit from cardioversion include those with AF lasting more than 1 year, LA enlargement, and recurrence while taking appropriate doses of antiarrhythmic agents who have recently undergone cardioversion.[16]

DEVICE THERAPY

In some patients with HF with AF, rate control can be difficult to achieve with medications. An ablation of the atrioventricular (AV) node/bundle of His with implantation of a permanent pacemaker may be useful as a form of rate control.[3,6,18] Chronic resynchronization therapy, often referred to as biventricular pacing, may be indicated for some patients in HF who also have AF, especially those with disease of the AV node, after AV node ablation, with systolic HF,[18] or if frequent ventricular pacing is anticipated (>40%) and will result in close to 100% ventricular pacing.

Patients in HF with reduced ejection fraction (EF) are at increased risk of ventricular arrhythmias and sudden cardiac death. An implantable cardioverter defibrillator (ICD) may be needed, especially those who have previously experienced ventricular tachycardia, ventricular fibrillation, unexplained syncope, and cardiac arrest. Coexisting AF can be problematic with an ICD, despite the optimization of device settings, such as tachycardia detection rates. Clearly, device reprogramming to minimize inappropriate shocks needs to be balanced with the risk of underdetection of arrhythmias.[3]

CATHETER ABLATION

It is well documented that atrial ectopic beats from the muscular sleeves of the pulmonary veins (PV) are one of the most common triggers of AF. In AF ablation, electrical disconnection of the PV from the LA is accomplished by ablation around the PV orifice, commonly called PV isolation.[14,17,19] These are created using radiofrequency or cryoablation is an invasive procedure typically performed in the electrophysiology or cardiac catheterization laboratory of a hospital for patients with AF. Radiofrequency energy generates alternating electrical current that destroys or ablates myocardial tissue, whereas cryoablation destroys tissues by freezing. Ablated tissue becomes nonconducting scar tissue. It has been shown to be safe and effective in patients with HF.[12] Outcomes for AF radiofrequency ablation are good compared with antiarrhythmic therapy.[17] Sinus rhythm can be obtained in 70% to 80% of patients following this procedure. In patients with HF, AF ablation has been associated with improvement of EF and improvement of HF symptoms.[15]

AF ablation requires a transseptal approach, crossing from the right atrium into the LA. It can be a lengthy procedure and it is often done using general anesthesia. It is done under fluoroscopy and echocardiographic guidance. Arrhythmia mapping is completed. Ablation catheters are placed and the tissue is treated. Frequent flushing of the ablation catheters is needed to cool the heat generated by radiofrequency. This additional volume must be considered in the patient with HF. Following the procedure, the patient is generally monitored overnight before being discharged home. Dull chest pain from inflammation caused by ablation usually resolves over a few days. The patient may continue to have some continued or intermittent arrhythmia. Anti-arrhythmic therapy may be continued while this resolves.[20]

Major complications can occur in up to 4.5% of procedures, including cardiac tamponade due to perforation, injury to phrenic nerve, esophageal injury, stroke, other atrial arrhythmias, vascular complications, and death. A late complication that can occur is PV stenosis. Recurrent AF is common in the first 3 months after the procedure (40%–50%). Because of this, anticoagulation is recommended for 2 months following ablation. Patients should be reevaluated within 3 to 4 months to assess outcome.[17] Repeat ablations may necessary.[11]

HYBRID ABLATION

A newer technique being done for AF is a hybrid approach: combining catheter-based and surgical techniques. An endocardial-epicardial ablation approach is less invasive, avoids the need for surgical incisions, lung deflation, and heart dissection. A transdiaphragmatic endoscopic approach is used to make epicardial lesions. Mapping and endocardial ablation is then done. Overall, this approach has been found to be safe and efficacious but is mostly done in patients without concomitant HF.[21]

SURGICAL ABLATION

Surgical ablation of AF has been available for several years and is commonly referred to as the maze procedure. It is open-heart surgical approach requiring cardiopulmonary bypass. Operative mortality is approximately 3%. Multiple incisions are placed within the atria, using radiofrequency, cryoablation, and/or laser, interrupting the reentry pathways and stopping the AF. This procedure is successful in most patients and can lead to improvements in EF, functional class, and quality of life.[12] Continuing enhancements have been made to this procedure resulting in less procedural morbidity and mortality.[22] Select patients may benefit from a thoracoscopic approach and modified maze procedure. Surgical ablation is typically considered in patients who are undergoing surgery for other cardiac conditions, such as the need for coronary artery bypass or valve repair/replacement surgery. Additionally, it may be considered in patients who have recurrent AF after more than one catheter ablation procedure and rhythm control is still indicated, especially if there is significant atrial remodeling with LA size exceeding 5 cm.[3]

LEFT ATRIAL APPENDAGE OCCLUSION

The LAA is the primary source for thromboembolism in AF. Exclusion or closure of the LAA, either with a device or during cardiac surgery, may be done for preventing stroke. Current devices in use include the Amplatzer Cardiac Plug (St Jude Medical, St Paul, MN), the Lariat (SentreHEART, Redwood City, CA), and The WATCHMAN device (Boston Scientific, Natick, MA). Surgical excision of the LAA may be considered in patients undergoing cardiac surgery for another reason.[9]

OTHER STRATEGIES

The renin-angiotensin-aldosterone system (RAAS) plays a role in the development of AF. Medications that provide RAAS blockade have been found to be beneficial in decreasing electrical and structural remodeling.[23] These agents include angiotensin-converting enzyme inhibitors and angiotensin receptor blockers.[1,14] Additionally, aldosterone antagonists, such as eplerenone (Inspra), may also prevent AF in HF patients.[23,24] Although its mechanism is not fully understood, statin therapy is associated with a decreased risk of incidence or recurrence of AF. Patients with untreated obstructive sleep apnea have a 25% greater chance of recurrent AF following ablation.[5,23] Treatment of obstructive sleep apnea has been noted to decrease risk of recurrent AF, after cardioversion and ablation; additional research is needed to better understand its role in primary prevention of AF.

SUMMARY

HF and AF are 2 major cardiovascular disorders on the rise worldwide that have great clinical and financial impact. They frequently coexist and increase the risk of morbidity and mortality. AF and HF share common mechanisms, and treatment strategies and therapies directed toward HF may protect against the occurrence of AF. The mainstays of the clinical approach to the HF and AF and patients remain optimal treatment of HF, anticoagulation, and rate or rhythm control. Clinical trials have failed to demonstrate a distinct advantage of sinus rhythm over optimal control of heart rate. In addition to various currently available rate or rhythm control medications, devices such as pacemakers and ICDs, and procedures such as cardioversion or ablation can be beneficial to many patients.

REFERENCES

1. Lubitz SA, Benjamin EJ, Ellinor PT. Atrial fibrillation in congestive heart failure. Heart Fail Clin 2010;6(2):187–200.
2. Ferreira JP, Santos M. Heart failure and atrial fibrillation: from basic science to clinical practice. Int J Mol Sci 2015;16:3133–47.
3. Havmöller R, Chugh SS. Atrial fibrillation in heart failure. Curr Heart Fail Rep 2012; 9:309–18.
4. Centers for Disease Control and Prevention. Division for Heart Disease and Stroke Protection. CDC. Available at: http://www.cdc.gov/dhdsp/data_statistics/index.htm. Accessed June 7, 2015.
5. Mozaffarian D, Benjamin EJ, Go AS, et al, on behalf of the American Heart Association Statistics Committee and Stroke Statistics Subcommittee. Heart disease and stroke statistics—2015 update: a report from the American Heart Association. Circulation 2015;131:e29–322.
6. Antar E, Jessup M, Callans DJ. Atrial fibrillation and heart failure: treatment considerations for a dual epidemic. Circulation 2009;119:2516–25.
7. Cheng A, Kumar K. Overview of atrial fibrillation. UptoDate. Available at: www.uptodate.com/contents/overview-of-atrial-fibrillation. Accessed May 27, 2015.
8. Iwasaki Y, Nishida K, Kato T, et al. Atrial fibrillation pathophysiology: implications for management. Circulation 2011;124:2264–74.
9. January CT, Wann LS, Alpert JS, et al. 2014 AHA/ACC/HRS guideline for the management of patients with atrial fibrillation: executive summary: a report of the American College of Cardiology/American Heart Association Task Force on Practice Guidelines and the Heart Rhythm Society. J Am Coll Cardiol 2014;64:2246–80.
10. Yancy CW, Jessup M, Bozkurt B, et al. 2013 ACCF/AHA guideline for the management of heart failure: a report of the American College of Cardiology Foundation/American Heart Association task force on practice guidelines. Circulation 2013;128:e240–327.
11. Aagaard P, Di Biase L, Natale A. Ablation of atrial arrhythmias in heart failure. Heart Fail Clin 2015;11:305–17.
12. Lardizabal JA, Deedwania PC. Atrial fibrillation in heart failure. Med Clin North Am 2012;96:987–1000.
13. Prasun MA. Providing best practice in the management of atrial fibrillation in the United States. J Cardiovasc Nurs 2012;27(5):445–56.
14. Sharma AK, Mansour M, Ruskin JN, et al. Atrial fibrillation and congestive heart failure. The Journal of Innovations in Cardiac Rhythm Management 2011;2:253–62.
15. Leong-Sit P, Tang ASL. Atrial fibrillation and heart failure: a bad combination. Curr Opin Cardiol 2015;30:161–7.
16. Naccarelli GV, Ganz LI, Manning WJ. Atrial fibrillation: cardioversion to sinus rhythm. UpToDate. Available at: www.uptodate.com/contents/atrial-fibrillation-cardioversion-to-sinus-rhythm. Accessed May 27, 2015.
17. Wazni Q, Wilkoff B, Saliba W. Catheter ablation for atrial fibrillation. N Engl J Med 2011;365:2296–304.
18. Saxon LA. Cardiac resynchronization therapy in atrial fibrillation. UpToDate. Available at: www.uptodate/contents/cardiac-resynchronication-theray-in-atrial-fibrillation. Accessed May 27, 2015.
19. Rabah A, Wazni O. Atrial fibrillation in heart failure: catheter and surgical interventional therapies. Heart Fail Rev 2014;9:325–30.
20. Zak J. Ablation to treat atrial fibrillation: beyond rhythm control. Crit Care Nurse 2010;30(6):68–79.

21. Trulock KM, Narayan SM, Piccini JP. Rhythm control in heart failure patients with atrial fibrillation. J Am Coll Cardiol 2014;64(7):710–21.
22. Thihalolipavan S, Morin DP. Atrial fibrillation and congestive heart failure. Heart Fail Clin 2014;10:305–18.
23. Wung SF. Atrial fibrillation in the elderly: management strategies to achieve performance measures. AACN Adv Crit Care 2014;25(3):205–12.
24. VanWagoner DR, Piccini JP, Albert CM, et al. Progress toward the prevention and treatment of atrial fibrillation: a summary of the Heart Rhythm Society research forum on the treatment and prevention of atrial fibrillation. Heart Rhythm 2015; 12:e5–29.

Hypertensive Crisis
A Review of Pathophysiology and Treatment

Deborah A. Taylor, PharmD

KEYWORDS

- Hypertensive urgency • Hypertensive emergency • Hypertensive crisis

KEY POINTS

- Treatment guidelines have been published by Joint National Committee (JNC) groups in an effort to reduce hypertension.
- Patients with hypertensive urgency may only need treatment with oral medications and can be safely discharged with close follow-up with a medical professional. Blood pressure in these patients will still be elevated above normal.
- Patients with hypertensive emergency require admission to intensive care units and administration of intravenous medications to safely reduce blood pressure levels. Blood pressure in these patients must be reduced over a period of time to avoid other medical crisis.
- The effects that hypertension has on vital the organs of the body has been shown to lead to other health issues in most patients.
- It is important for medical practitioners to have a working knowledge of medications for hypertensive crisis.

INTRODUCTION

According to the Centers for Disease Control and Prevention, approximately 70 million American adults (29%) have hypertension and only about half (52%) have their blood pressure (BP) under control.[1,2] When uncontrolled over a time span of years, hypertension can lead to damage of vital organs, namely the cardiovascular, neurologic, and renal systems. Many medications are on the market to treat patients with hypertension. Knowledge of these agents, their characteristics, and their proper use helps to decrease the damage to organs that ultimately will result in an increased cost burden to the health care system.

Guidelines for treatment of hypertension were changed in late 2013 with the publication of the 2014 evidence-based guideline for the management of high BP in adults

Disclosures: None.
Department of Pharmacy and Clinical Nutrition, Grady Health System, 80 Jesse Hill Jr Drive SE, Atlanta, GA 30303, USA
E-mail address: dtaylor@gmh.edu

from the panel members appointed to the Eighth Joint National Committee (JNC8).[3] Treatment modalities were now based on age, race, and the presence of diabetes mellitus or chronic kidney disease.

Despite these recommendations and others, however, clinicians continue to see many patients with undiagnosed and uncontrolled hypertension. Because the choice of medical therapy is crucial, through PubMed searches this article reviews the pathophysiology of hypertensive crisis and the treatment choices currently available.

DEFINITIONS

Hypertensive crisis by definition is divided into 2 categories: hypertensive urgency or hypertensive emergency.[2,4–6] Both groups present with severely elevated BP, but the differences lie in the presence of target organ damage (TOD) (seen only in hypertensive emergency) and the treatment options (**Fig. 1**).

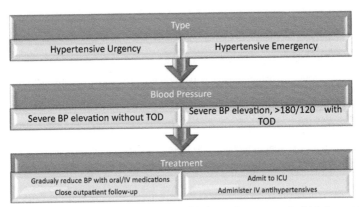

Fig. 1. Hypertensive crisis. BP, blood pressure; ICU, intensive care unit; IV, intravenous; TOD, target organ damage.

CLINICAL PRESENTATION
Hypertensive Urgency

Patients will present with elevated BP greater than 180/120 mm Hg, without signs of TOD. Presenting symptoms may include headache, shortness of breath, anxiety, and epistaxis.[7]

Hypertensive Emergency

Patients will present with elevated BP greater than 180/120 mm Hg, and will show signs of TOD (**Box 1**).

When a patient presents with hypertensive crisis, several things should be done as soon as possible, including mental status checks, continuous monitoring of BP, and an electrocardiogram to ascertain heart rate and rhythm. The physician should obtain a medical history noting the length and extent of the presenting symptoms, and a review of all current medications (prescription and nonprescription), and ask questions to determine medication compliance and recreational drug use.[6–8] Close attention should paid to those patients with comorbid disease states and effects on the neurologic, renal, and cardiovascular systems.

> **Box 1**
> **Signs of target organ damage seen in hypertensive emergency**
>
> *Cardiac*
> - Aortic dissection
> - Heart failure/left ventricular hypertension
> - Acute pulmonary edema
> - Myocardial ischemia/unstable angina
>
> *Renal*
> - Acute/chronic renal disease
> - Hematuria
>
> *Neurologic*
> - Cerebral vascular accident
> - Intracerebral hemorrhage
> - Headache
> - Confusion
> - Visual loss
> - Hypertensive encephalopathy
>
> *Ophthalmic*
> - Retinopathy
>
> Data from Refs.[7,8,15]

PATHOPHYSIOLOGY

Armed with the knowledge of the many causes of hypertension and hypertensive crisis, this article initially reviews normal autoregulation of blood flow.[9–11]

BP is the pressure or tension exerted by the blood as it circulates through the arterial vessels, and is expressed in mm Hg (millimeters of mercury). As seen by the following equation, BP is a product of cardiac output (CO) and total peripheral resistance (TPR).

$$BP = CO \times TPR$$

Factors that contribute to hypertension include, but are not limited to, malfunctions in the humoral system (ie, the renin-angiotensin-aldosterone system) and the neuronal and autoregulatory systems.

Autoregulation is defined as the intrinsic ability of an organ to maintain a constant blood flow despite changes in perfusion pressure (arterial minus venous pressure, $P_A - P_V$). When perfusion pressure decreases to an organ, blood flow (F) initially decreases, but returns toward normal levels over the next few minutes. This autoregulatory response occurs in the absence of neural and hormonal influences and therefore is intrinsic to that organ. Autoregulation occurs normally in response to hypoperfusion to the brain, heart, and kidneys.

In the equation displayed in **Fig. 2**, when perfusion pressure initially decreases, blood flow F decreases because of the relationship between pressure, flow, and resistance.[12]

Autoregulation helps to maintain normal blood flow to vital organs while maintaining a homeostatic BP.

$$F = \frac{(P_A - P_V)}{R}$$

Fig. 2. Autoregulation equation. (*From* Klabunde RE. Cardiovascular physiology concepts. Available at: http://www.cvphysiology.com. Accessed July, 2015; with permission.)

Fig. 3 shows the effects of suddenly reducing perfusion pressure from 100 to 70 mm Hg in a vascular bed without autoregulation. There is a decrease in blood flow and an increase in vascular resistance. In organs with autoregulation, after the initial decrease in perfusion pressure and flow, the flow will gradually increase as the vasculature dilates and resistance decreases (*red lines* in **Fig. 3**). After a few minutes, the flow will achieve a new steady-state level very close to normal.[9]

Failure of this autoregulatory response is seen in hypertensive crisis. Resistance, and BP, will continue to increase with loss of the autoregulation.

ETIOLOGY

Most patients who present with hypertensive crisis usually have a history of hypertension. The following list includes some of the commonly suggested causes of hypertensive crisis:

Pregnancy
    Preeclampsia, eclampsia
Medications
    Compliance
    Sudden withdrawal of medications, especially β-blockers, clonidine
    Therapeutic inertia: providers' failure to increase therapy when treatment goals
        are unmet[13]
Drug interactions

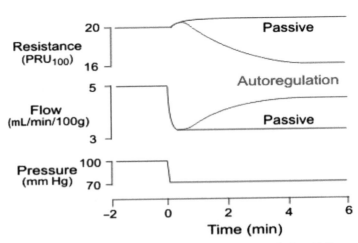

Fig. 3. Effects of perfusion pressure reduction without autoregulation. PRU_{100}, peripheral resistance units per 100 g tissue. (*From* Klabunde RE. Cardiovascular physiology concepts. Available at: http://www.cvphysiology.com. Accessed July, 2015; with permission.)

Table 1
Parenteral infusions for rapid blood pressure control in hypertensive emergencies

Drug	Dosage	Onset (min)	Duration	Comments
Nitrates				
Sodium nitroprusside	0.5 μg/kg/min, increase 0.5 μg/kg/min every 20–60 min	<2	1–10 min	Black-box warning.[c] Max. dose 10 μg/kg/min. Caution when used with other antihypertensives
Nitroglycerin	5 μg/min, increase by 5 μg/min every 3–5 min up to 20 μg/min	Immediate	3–5 min	Ensure adequate hydration. Use with caution in head trauma, avoid if recent use of Viagra (24 h) or Cialis (48 h)
Calcium-Channel Blockers				
Clevidipine	1–2 mg/h initially, usual dose ~4–6 mg/h	2–4	5–15 min	Titration–may double every 90 s to goal BP. Every 1–2 mg/h increase equals ~2–4 mm Hg SBP reduction
Nicardipine	5 mg/h initially, increasing by 2.5 mg/h every 15 min to max. 15 mg/h	10	≤8 h	Consider reducing at rate of 3 mg/h after response is achieved
Dopamine-1 Agonist				
Fenoldopam	0.1–0.3 μg/kg/min, increasing by 0.05–0.1 μg/kg/min every 15 min to target BP	10	1 h	Use for short-term reduction of BP for up to 48 h. Use low initial dose to prevent reflex tachycardia
Adrenergic-Blocking Agents				
Labetalol	Bolus 10–20 mg, then infusion 2 mg/min initially, titrating to response. Max. 6 mg/min	2–5	2–18 h (based on single and subsequent doses)	Do not withdraw abruptly
Esmolol	Varies by situation	2–10 (quickest time if loading dose given)	10–30 min	Used also for intra- and postoperative hypertension

(continued on next page)

Table 1
(continued)

Drug	Dosage	Onset (min)	Duration	Comments
Other Agents				
Hydralazine	Preeclampsia or eclampsia: 5 mg/dose, then 5–10 mg every 20–30 min as needed Hypertension: IV, 10–20 mg/dose every 4–6 h as needed. May increase to 40 mg/dose. Change to oral as soon as possible	5–20	1–4 h, depending on whether patient is a fast or slow acetylator[a]	Use for hypertension secondary to preeclampsia or eclampsia
Enalaprilat	IV dose is 1.25 mg 6 h over a 5-min period	15–30	6–12 h	Slow onset, long duration, frequent dosing (every 6 h), used when patient cannot take oral
Phentolamine	5–20 mg for hypertensive crisis, 5 mg IV 1–2 h Surgery due to pheochromocytoma: 5 mg (max. dose) 1–2 h before procedure, repeat as needed every 2–4 h until hypertension controlled	Immediate	15–30 min	Hypertension associated with pheochromocytoma[b]

Abbreviations: BP, blood pressure; IV, intravenous; max., maximum; SBP, systolic blood pressure.

[a] Acetylator: an organism capable of metabolic acetylation. Those animals that differ in their inherited ability to metabolize certain drugs, for example, isoniazid and hydralazine, are termed fast or slow acetylators.

[b] Pheochromocytoma: a tumor of the adrenal glands. Symptoms include headache, sweating, palpitations, and elevated BP (http://medical-dictionary.thefreedictionary.com).

[c] A cautionary label for all therapeutic agents and/or products and relevant literature that the FDA regards as being hazardous to health if incorrectly administered (http://medical-dictionary.thefreedictionary.com).

Data from Refs.[5,6,11,12,15,16]

Box 2
Most common side effects of hypertension drugs

Nitroprusside

Acute coronary syndrome (ACS), aortic dissection, blood pressure control after bypass surgery

Adverse events (AE): headache, palpitations, bradycardia, cyanide toxicity, hypothyroidism, methemoglobinemia

Use is limited because of the black-box warning[a] "contains cyanide molecules that can accumulate in the body in renal and hepatic failure patients." Nitroprusside should be administered at the same time as a longer-acting antihypertensive medication so that the duration of treatment with nitroprusside can be minimized.

Nitroglycerin

ACS, preeclampsia

AE: reflex tachycardia, headache, methemoglobinemia

Clevidipine

ACS, postoperative hypertensive emergency

AE: reflex tachycardia, nausea/vomiting, headache, hypotension

Note: formulation contains soy and egg. Watch for allergic reaction in affected patients.

Nicardipine

ACS

AE: flushing, tachycardia, palpitations, pulmonary edema, nausea/vomiting

Fenoldopam

AE: headache, electrocardiogram (ECG) changes, hypotension, tachycardia, nausea/vomiting, xerostomia

Labetalol

Aortic dissection

AE: bradycardia, pulmonary edema, heart block

Esmolol

Aortic dissection

AE: headache, hypotension, wheezing, ECG changes, hypotension, bradycardia

Hydralazine

AE: edema, hypotension

Enalaprilat

Heart failure, hypertension when oral administration is not feasible

AE: hypotension, cough. Watch for signs of angioedema

Phentolamine

To counteract the effects of hypertension caused by catecholamine (occurs in pheochromocytoma, monoamine oxidase inhibitor interactions, cocaine or amphetamine use)

AE: hypotension, tachycardia, arrhythmias

[a] A black box warning indicates that medical studies show that the drug carries a considerable risk of serious or even life threatening adverse effects. The US Food and Drug Administration (FDA) may ask pharmaceutical companies to place a black-box warning on the labeling of a prescription drug, or in literature describing it. It is the strongest warning that the FDA requires.
Data from Refs.[5,6,11,12,14–16]

Monoamine oxidase inhibitors
Recreational drug use: increased release of catecholamines
  Cocaine
  Amphetamines
Head trauma
Postoperative presentation

PHARMACOLOGIC TREATMENT APPROACH
Hypertensive Urgency

For patients who present with hypertensive urgency, the goal is not to reduce BP to normal.[5,6,11,12,14–17] Patients may be under observation for a few hours with medical therapy that may include the restart or titration of home/previous medications. Patients must be monitored for signs of TOD and altered mental status.

Hypertensive Emergency

Patients are admitted to the intensive care unit for medical treatment with parenteral antihypertensives. Close monitoring of these patients is essential, as arterial lines are frequently used for infusion of medications (**Table 1**).

Regarding which drugs should be used and the potential adverse effects to watch out for, it should be borne in mind that all agents can cause hypotension. **Box 2** should be used only as a guide.

SUMMARY

It is important to evaluate and treat patients newly diagnosed with hypertension with proper medications and follow-up to prevent the progression of uncontrolled hypertension to hypertensive urgency or emergency. The prompt recognition of a hypertensive emergency at triage with the appropriate diagnostic tests will lead to the adequate reduction of BP, ameliorating the incidence of negative consequences. Adequate treatment will help to alleviate the progression of disease and improve long-term outcomes.[1]

REFERENCES

1. Rodriguez MA, Kumar SK, De Caro M. Hypertensive crisis. Cardiol Rev 2010; 18(2):102–7.
2. Hypertension. Available at: http://www.cdc.gov/nchs/fastats/default.htm. Accessed July, 2015.
3. James PA, Oparil S, Carter BL, et al. 2014 evidence-based guideline for the management of high blood pressure in adults: report from the panel members appointed to the Eighth Joint National Committee (JNC 8). JAMA 2014;311(5):507–20.
4. Nwankwo T, Yoon SS, Burt V, et al. Hypertension among adults in the US: National Health and Nutrition Examination Survey, 2011-2012. NCHS data brief, no. 133. Hyattsville (MD): National Center for Health Statistics, Centers for Disease Control and Prevention, US Dept of Health and Human Services; 2013.
5. Morrison A, Vijayan A. Hypertension. In: The Washington manual of medical therapeutics. 32nd edition. Philadephia: Lippincott Williams & Wilkins; 2007. p. 102–18.
6. Tuncel M, Ram V. Hypertensive emergencies. Am J Cardiovasc Drugs 2003;3(1): 21–31.

7. McKinnon M, O'Neill J. Hypertension in the emergency department: treat now, later, or not at all. Emerg Med Pract 2010;12:6.
8. ClinicalAdvisor. Stat Consult: hypertensive emergency/hypertensive urgency. 2012. Available at: www.clinicaladvisor.com. Accessed July 2015.
9. Klabunde R. Cardiovascular physiology concepts. 2nd edition. 2011. Available at: www.cvphysiology.com, www.cvpharmacology.com. Accessed July, 2015.
10. Available at: www.heart.org/Conditions/HighBloodPressure. Accessed July, 2015.
11. Dipiro J, Talbert R, Saseen JJ, et al. Pharmacotherapy. A pathological approach. 7th edition. p. 141–71.
12. Available at: druginfo.com. Accessed August, 2015.
13. Okonofua EC, Simpson KN, Jesri A, et al. Therapeutic inertia is an impediment to achieving the healthy people 2010 blood pressure control goals. Hypertension 2006;47:345–51.
14. Available at: http://www.uptodate.com. Accessed August, 2015.
15. Varon J, Marik P. Management of hypertensive crises. Crit Care 2003;7(5): 374–84.
16. Tulman DB, Stawicki SP, Papadimos TJ, et al. Advances in management of acute hypertension: a concise review. Discov Med 2012;13(72):375–83. Accessed July, 2015.
17. Slama M, Modeliar SS. Hypertension in the intensive care unit. Curr Opin Cardiol 2006;21:279–87. Lippincott Williams & Wilkins.

Hemodynamics of Acute Right Heart Failure in Mechanically Ventilated Patients with Acute Respiratory Distress Syndrome

Barbara McLean, MN, RN, CCNS-BC, NP-BC, CCRN, FCCM

KEYWORDS

- Right heart dysfunction • Cor pulmonale • Pulmonary hypertension

KEY POINTS

- The study of right ventricular (RV) dysfunction in intensively ill, mechanically ventilated, and in particular patients diagnosed with ARDS is a new field.
- The RV is significantly susceptible to an increase in afterload (pulmonary vascular resistance), decreased contractility, and primary or secondary alterations in preload (volume and compliance) when challenged with high intrapulmonary pressures.
- In the face of hypoxemic hypoxia, high mean airway pressures, increased shunt, and aggressive volume resuscitation, one should question the validity of monitoring the pulmonary artery (PA) pressures and cardiac output/cardiac index as indicative of isolated LV failure.
- For patients with diagnosed RV dysfunction and ARDS, echocardiogram needs to be used to evaluate the effects of positive pressure on RF performance and LV filling.

INTRODUCTION

In critically ill patients with circulatory shock, the role of the left ventricle (LV) has long been appreciated and the object of measurement and therapeutic targeting. The right ventricle (RV), because of its thinner walls and often nonspecific ejection targets, is often undervisualized and overlooked. Generally, the RV operates passively, with little work or tension required to support the ejection of the diastolic volume. A loss of ventricular wall compliance (diastolic dysfunction) results in an alteration in the normal pressure-volume relationship. Traditional right heart filling indices (right atrial [RA] pressure and/or central venous pressure [CVP]) may increase because of the decreasing compliance. This elevation is frequently incorrectly interpreted as overall

Division of Critical Care, Grady Health System, Atlanta, GA, USA
E-mail address: bamclean@mindspring.com

Crit Care Nurs Clin N Am 27 (2015) 449–467
http://dx.doi.org/10.1016/j.cnc.2015.08.002
0899-5885/15/$ – see front matter © 2015 Elsevier Inc. All rights reserved.

volume overload or indicative of LV dysfunction, when left ventricular end diastolic volume may actually be critical (secondarily to the RV volume alterations). The elevation in RV filling pressures may also indicate significant obstruction to flow through the pulmonary vascular bed (from positive pressure ventilation or pulmonary embolism). Pulmonary vascular dysfunction in acute respiratory distress syndrome (ARDS) is particularly related to the effects of a mean airway pressure strategy (positive end-expiratory pressure [PEEP], high opening airway pressures) and may contribute to acute cor pulmonale (ACP).[1–3]

The study of RV dysfunction in intensively ill, mechanically ventilated, and in particular, patients diagnosed with ARDS is a new field and knowledge has been built based on the comparison of arterial and pulmonary arterial pressures and calculated cardiac outputs,[4–6] and echocardiographic proof of significant effects on the RV.[3] This article presents a concise clinical perspective on acute respiratory distress and progressive positive mean airway pressure strategies that may induce ACP and RV failure.

ACUTE RIGHT VENTRICULAR FAILURE

The right heart, comprising the right atrium and RV, ejects about 75% of the total volume received by the end of diastole (RV end diastolic volume typically estimated with CVP) into the pulmonary circulation. The RV normally operates below its unstressed volume (ie, increasing filling volume does not raise pressure because the RV is relatively compliant under normal circumstances) and therefore the measured RA pressure may not reflect true volume load.[7] Fig. 1A highlights the filling pressures of RV and LV and the corresponding diastolic pressures in the exiting arteries (pulmonary and aorta). The compliant pulmonary vasculature is typically characterized by low resistance, therefore the work of the RV is significantly less than that of the LV, requiring little tension or muscular development to overcome that afterload.

In critically ill patients, the RV is significantly susceptible to an increase in afterload (pulmonary vascular resistance), decreased contractility, and primary or secondary alterations in preload (volume and compliance) (Fig. 1B). All three of these factors may be significantly affected by the introduction of positive pressure ventilation strategies focused on the mean airway pressure with little to no regard to the compromise placed

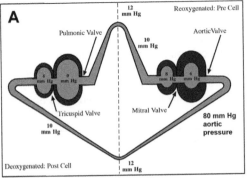
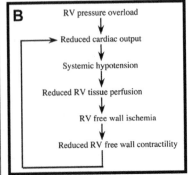

Fig. 1. (A) Visualizing the normal pressure relationships associated with right and left ventricular function. (B) The pathway to right ventricular dysfunction.

on RV function.[8,9] Acute right heart failure is traditionally defined as the association of RV dilatation with a paradoxic septal motion at end-systole.[10]

Early studies have supported incidence of RV dysfunction in the trauma/shock/septic shock population possibly related to right heart volume overload in conjunction with acute pulmonary hypertension.[11] The displacement of the intraventricular septum toward the LV causes a significant increase in the filling pressure or pressure required to fill the LV and is often evaluated as the pulmonary capillary wedge pressure (PCW) or pulmonary arterial occlusion pressure. The filling pressure elevation is often interpreted as an indicator of primary left heart failure. Although this may be the case, it is essential to recall that unlike the LV, which is uniquely designed to adjust contractile tension to volume and resistance loads, the RV is architecturally incapable of acute adjustment to load variables (preload and afterload). In the critical care environment, careful attention should be paid to the effects of positive pressure ventilation strategies, particularly in the ARDS population. **Fig. 2** highlights the effects of increasing mean airway pressure strategies (ie, PEEP, airway pressure release ventilation, prolonged inspiratory time).

Pressure Monitoring

RA and left atrial (LA) pressures are used to determine the relationship of ventricular filling to valvular function, ventricular compliance, and volume load. The pressure gradient of vein to atria through valve to ventricle determines the efficacy of filling.

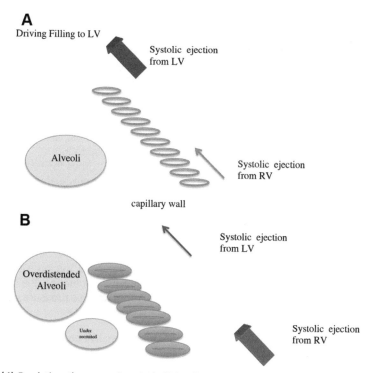

Fig. 2. (*A*) Depicting the normal endothelial cellular wall that separates alveoli from blood flow and the proportional pressures of left (*red*) and right (*blue*) heart. (*B*) Depicting the effects of noncompliant pulmonary vasculature that separates alveoli from blood flow and the proportional pressures of left (*red*) and right (*blue*) heart.

The normal RV filling pressure is close to atmosphere (760 mm Hg), which is tradition-ally known as "zero." The RA filling pressure is typically 2 to 8 mm Hg, which provides enough of a gradient to maximize RV filling. The CVP is slightly higher, at 4 to 10 mm Hg, and supports the filling of the right atria, which then maximizes RV filling. This gradient of pressure is normally enhanced by alterations in the intrathoracic pressure during spontaneous (unassisted) inspiration.[12] Normal, nonassisted ventilation is pro-moted by a pressure drop in the intrathoracic cavity below atmospheric pressure (negative inspiratory pressure) but varies with every breath. This drop in pressure is communicated across the myocardial surface, basically increasing the RV diameter and dropping the RV pressure below "zero." The negative pressure gradient supports the increasing volume loading of the RV, while maintaining a fairly constant filling pres-sure. The filling of the RV is effectively maintained as long as the right-sided valves are competent and mobile, the RV is compliant, the septal wall is in place, the patient is euvolemic, and there is an increasing negative pressure during inspiration.

The normal LV filling pressure is close to 8 mm Hg (see **Fig. 1**A). The higher filling pressure of the LV is directly related to the tensile and muscular properties of the LV as opposed to the RV. The LA pressure is around 4 to 8 mm Hg, which along with atrial contraction at the end of ventricular filling typically provides enough of a gradient to almost maximize LV filling.

The pulmonary venous pressure is slightly higher at 6 to 12 mm Hg and reflects the pressure gradient required to fill to fill the LA. Pulmonary capillary pressure is still higher (8–12 mm Hg). This pressure gradient (filling) begins at the alveolar capillary level and is activated on diastole, when the mitral valve is open (see **Fig. 1**A). Because low resistance and high compliance characterize the pulmonary vasculature, typical pulmonary artery pressures are quite low, normally around 25/10 mm Hg. The low resistance of the pulmonary system is enhanced by the alterations in LV compliance and pressure changes during inspiration and exhalation. During negative pressure inspiration, the systemic venovolume is literally "sucked" into the RV, increasing vol-ume loading and maintaining a fairly constant filling pressure. During exhalation, that volume is pushed by the more positive pressure into the LA and LV. The filling of the LV is effectively maintained as long as the left-sided valves are competent and mobile, the LV is compliant, the septal wall is in place, the patient is euvolemic, and has no signif-icant changes to the pressure gradient developed during inspiration.

The pulmonary artery catheter was initially developed to improve the evaluation and treatment of the cardiac patient in critical care. The basic theory was that the catheter would assist in the evaluation of the dynamic flow of blood from the pulmonic valve through the pulmonary vascular vault to the end point of venous flow, the LV. As the LV became noncompliant the left atria, pulmonary veins, right atria, and central veins would become engorged and noncompliant themselves.[12] The measured pressures (measuring the relationship of volume and chamber compliance) would rise. Histori-cally, these pressure measurements became synonymous with volume regulation, with little to no regard for the loss of compliance, valvular competence, the compres-sion of the pericardial sac, septal deviation, or evolution in positive pressure ventilation strategies designed to "open the lung."

Right Atrial Pressure (Right Atrial or Central Venous Pressure) and Pulmonary Arteriole Occlusion Pressure

In shock there are often several conditions that affect the ventricular filling pressures. First there is the evident arterial hypovolemia. If the patient experienced essential vol-ume loss on the street and/or in the operating room, they experience profound volume deficit. That deficit encourages systemic vasoconstriction, which together with the hypoperfusion elicits tissue hypoxia. The tissue hypoxia stimulates a systemic inflammatory response, most particularly encouraging neutrophil mobilization. The neutrophils may sequester in the lung and if this process is unchecked, lung injury may occur because alveoli become dysfunctional (atelectatic and/or inflamed) and the pulmonary capillaries constrict, increasing the tension that the RV must generate to mobilize volume. This increase in tension can be seen as a significant increase in RA pressure, which often equals or exceeds the LA pressure. In addition, the pulmonary arterial pressures increase significantly, often mimicking the systemic pressures in this patient. As the volume to the right heart increases, primarily caused by resuscitation efforts, the septal wall deviates to the LV, causing the chamber to be smaller and less compliant. The occlusion pressure (PCW) increases; however, systemic pressure drops. More volume is then given to resuscitate the pressure. The patient presents with profound venohypervolemia and significant arterial hypovolemia.

Traditionally, the response to this conundrum is to give more volume, diuresis, and possibly a vasoconstrictor, which may further exacerbate the initial problem. The patient who is ventilated may exhibit refractory hypoxia, which often necessitates increasing air trapping with mechanical (prolonged inspiratory time, shortened expiratory time) or circuit (applied at the ventilator) PEEP.

OXYGENATION

The starting and ending point of invasive and noninvasive hemodynamics is gas exchange: external at the alveoli/capillary (A-C) interface, and internal at the capillary/cell interface. The arterial blood gas, in combination with selected chemistry variables, provides direct information about ventilation and oxygenation and indirect information about tissue metabolism, tissue perfusion, and cellular or internal respiration (tissue oxygenation).

External Respiration

External respiration is profoundly affected by alveolar distention, Pao_2, and blood flow through the pulmonary vault, hemoglobin, and the distance between the alveolus and capillary. The relationship of gas in alveolus to gas in the blood is measured as $AaDo_2$, and most easily by the proportional ratio of Pao_2 to the FiO_2 (P/F ratio) (**Table 1**). The importance of evaluating the relationship of arterial oxygen, Pao_2, with the assumed alveolar gas is of significant concern in all patients, but particularly in ventilated patients with ARDS. If alveolar sacs are distendable and compliant, the airways are open, and the patient is breathing appropriate volumes, gas is delivered to the alveolar

Table 1
Gas to blood relationships measured by alveoli (hypothetical) and measured arterial oxygen

Measure	Formula	Normal	Abnormal	Shunt
Aa DO_2	FiO_2 (Baro Pressure − Water Vapor) − $PaCO_2$/RQ = A gas 0.21 (760 mm Hg − 47) − 40/0.8 = 149.7 − 50 = 99.7 $PAo_2 = 99.7$ Pao_2 = measured from ABG $PAo_2 - Pao_2 = AaDO_2$	<FiO_2 10–20	>FiO_2 >20	>150
P to F	Pao_2/FiO_2 100/0.21 = 476	>400	<200	<200 if FiO_2 >0.4

sacs. If the blood flow by the alveolar sacs is constant and unobstructed, gas exchange takes place. The gas at high concentration in the alveoli (oxygen) moves into the blood, the gas at high concentration in the blood (carbon dioxide) moves into the alveolus. Therefore the relationship of gas exchange at the A-C interface is measured by the correlation of theoretic gas in the alveolus, PaO_2 (assumed by percent of inhaled gas that is oxygenated), to the measured dissolved gas in the blood, PaO_2.

The P/F ratio and the $AaDo_2$ are estimates of intrapulmonary shunting (Qs/Q_T), which is affected by the tidal volume, respiratory rate, resistance of the airways, alveolar distention, and blood flow past the alveolar sacs, and the distance between the alveoli and the capillary. The acute heart failure patient often exhibits a combination of alveolar destruction, inflammatory changes, pulmonary edema, alveolar collapse, and reduced pulmonary blood flow states. These conditions are referred to as acute lung injury, ARDS, and/or atelectasis. The failure of uptake of oxygen is evaluated by an extremely wide $AaDo_2$ and low P/F ratio in a ventilated patient on fraction of inspired oxygen greater than 0.40 (40%) and is judged by amount of distending airway pressures required to maintain acceptable dissolved oxygen states. This type of gas exchange failure is referred to as intrapulmonary shunt; that is, blood moves past the alveoli without being oxygenated, despite aggressive ventilator support.

The uptake of oxygen at the A-C interface determines the amount of oxygen available to deliver to the cell. The largest portion of oxygen in the blood is transported bound to hemoglobin and is best evaluated by the oxyhemoglobin on the arterial blood gas. In most institutions, this is trended by the pulse oximeter, which gives an approximation of the saturation of hemoglobin with oxygen (but tells nothing about the hemoglobin level, the more important concept in DO_2). Oxyhemoglobin provides an ever-ready reservoir of oxygen for the usable state, dissolved, in the blood. Usable oxygen is known as PaO_2. Therefore the role of hemoglobin is to keep the PaO_2 constant at the cellular level. Essentially, the higher the oxyhemoglobin, or arterial oxygen saturation (SaO_2), the higher is the PaO_2. This gives rise to the well-known oxyhemoglobin disassociation curve (**Fig. 3**). This curve shows the relationship of oxyhemoglobin (reservoir of oxygen, SaO_2) to the usable oxygen (dissolved, PaO_2). All this relationship shows at this juncture is the availability of oxygen in the arterial bed, or to the cells.

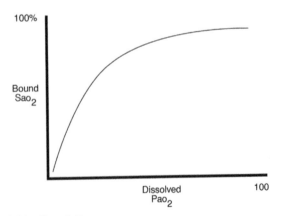

Fig. 3. Oxyhemoglobin dissociation curve.

AaDo$_2$, Sao$_2$, Pao$_2$, and P/F ratio evaluate the efficiency of A-C gas exchange, which in this population may be profoundly affected. The common tools Sao$_2$, Pao$_2$, AaDo$_2$, and P/F ratio all evaluate A-C gas exchange and oxygen availability, not usability.

Internal (Tissue Respiration)

Compensation in shock

The common underlying mechanism of shock no matter the cause is oxygen deficiency: cellular hypoxia, ischemia, and/or anoxia. This deficiency promotes a response heralded by increased circulating catecholamines and results in a compensatory increase in oxygen delivery (hallmarked by increasing heart rate, increased stroke volume, vasoconstriction of arterial and venous beds) and an increase in the proportionate use of oxygen (consumption divided by delivery). The resulting increase in venous return (affecting preload), vascular responses (altering afterload), and the increased output demands (affecting activation and contractility) may significantly alter the temporal myocardial balance of systole to diastole, the demand for high-energy phosphate bonds, and the resulting increase in myocardial oxygen consumption. The untoward demand for cardiac compensation in the patient with shock may be exacerbated and/or limited by true hypovolemia (affecting stroke volume) and/or inflammation or septic shock, which may significantly affect the vascular tone while increasing demands for oxygen delivery.

To evaluate usability of oxygen, it is vital to look at cellular indices of tissue oxygenation. These indicators include saturated hemoglobin (Svo$_2$), base excess, serum lactate, intramucosal pH, and various methods of imaging at the cellular level.

Because oxyhemoglobin provides an ever-ready reservoir of oxygen at the cellular level, it makes intuitive sense that evaluation of postcellular oxyhemoglobin would be telling in regards to cell function. Svo$_2$ measures the oxyhemoglobin reservoir after cellular uptake of dissolved oxygen and subsequent release of oxygen from the hemoglobin to keep dissolved (usable state) constant. This is a fairly global indicator of oxygen use at the cellular level, because Svo$_2$ is measured in the pulmonary artery after all blood has returned to the right heart and "mixed." In the patient with trauma or shock, one of the initial compensations is to shunt blood from low oxygen requiring organs and cells to the "essential" or high oxygen requiring organs and cells. As blood is shunted, peripheral pressures become more indicative of the loss of compliance of the arteries and less meaningful in terms of blood flow dynamics. The mixing of blood in the RA/RV/PA premixed venous measurement ensures that a global indicator reflects global oxygen use.

The comparison of Sao$_2$ with Svo$_2$ evaluates the global use of oxygen at the tissue level. If the tissues require greater oxygen because of hypermetabolism (pain, fever, acidosis), the oxyhemoglobin releases more to the dissolved state, causing a shift to the right (**Fig. 4**) or a decreased return of Svo$_2$. If the tissues require less oxygen or perfusion/extraction deficits are such that tissues are unable to use oxygen, the hemoglobin does not dissociate the oxygen, causing a shift to the left, or an increase in Svo$_2$ (**Fig. 5**).

The indicators of acidosis affect the circulating acid neutralizers approximated by calculate bicarbonate and/or base. Normal base is 0, with a range of +2 to -2. When base is in deficit (>−2), one must assume that circulating acid has increased. The most common reasons for an increase in circulating acid are (1) renal failure (validate with blood-urea-nitrogen and creatinine (Cr)), (2) ketosis (validate with history and blood sugar), (3) hyperchloremia (chloride levels <105), and (4) lactic acidosis (hypoperfusion) (**Fig. 6**).

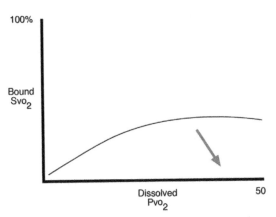

Fig. 4. Shift to the right of the oxyhemoglobin dissociation curve. Cells need it and they can get it.

The failure is at the cellular level: despite compensatory increases in oxygen delivery, the cells have a metabolic failure and are unable to extract oxygen, convert lactate to pyruvate, and therefore exhibit oxygen extraction failure and lactic acidosis. The patient might exhibits signs of sympathetic resistance, shock adrenal function, renal failure, and respiratory failure. The moment of truth arrives when the patient suffers cardiac failure from overcompensation, increases in myocardial oxygen demand, and inability to extract oxygen.

COMPENSATION

In shock (decrease in preload and decreased oxygen-carrying capacity) and profound systemic inflammatory response syndrome (profound inflammatory response resulting in hypermetabolism and vascular blood flow alterations), two compensatory mechanisms are evident in diagnosis: attempts to increase oxygen delivery (eg, an increase in heart rate and respiratory rate) and an increase in oxygen consumption.

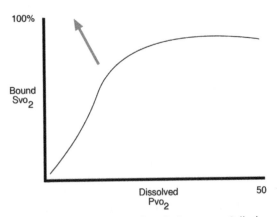

Fig. 5. Shift to the left of the oxyhemoglobin dissociation curve. Cells do not need it or need it but cannot get it.

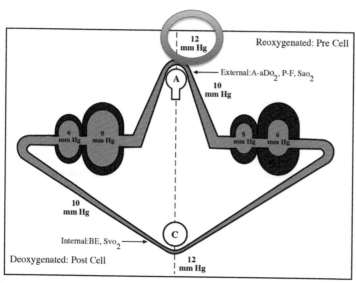

Fig. 6. Measurements of tissue oxygenation and the implementation of PEEP.

The proportionate consumption of oxygen to the delivery of oxygen, or oxygen extraction, is key in this condition. As shock, inflammation, and septicemia progress, the oxygen extraction becomes proportionately lower as the delivery of oxygen continues to increase. To support the demand, filling and ejection phases must be optimized. Both diastole and systole are active, energy-requiring processes with diastole more sensitive to a reduction in the available energy supply. The high demand may cause an uncoupling of the oxygen supply-demand relationship. Impaired relaxation results in decreased ventricular compliance that may result in increased PCW and CVPs. With reduced cardiac compliance, the filling pressures are not adequate indices of the volume status of the heart. Treatment regimens based on the assumption that elevated filling pressures indicate an elevated volume status may result in a reduction of the volume status and further cardiac decompensation.

Inadequate oxygen delivery or extraction may present as a failure of the myocardium to relax quickly and in an organized fashion. Relaxation failure causes increased resistance to filling (decreased compliance) and concomitantly causes filling pressures to rise. As compliance decreases, myocardial filling also decreases, which may result in suboptimal cardiac output, although the indices of systolic function (cardiac output/cardiac index) may not be below normal range. In keeping with Starling's law, the elevated filling pressures reflecting loss of compliance result in increased hydrostatic pressure, systemic and pulmonary venous congestion, and fluid extravasation. The filling pressures become more reflective of resistance to ventricular filling (loss of compliance) rather than volume.

Acute Cor Pulmonale

In the face of hypoxemic hypoxia, high mean airway pressures, increased shunt, and aggressive volume resuscitation, one should question the validity of monitoring the PA pressures and cardiac output/index as indicative of isolated LV failure. The thin-walled RV is much more sensitive to increases in afterload than the LV, making it vulnerable to systolic failure in disease states that raise RV afterload, a condition known as ACP. Acute RV dysfunction after cardiac surgery is associated with mortality rates of 80%.[13]

ARDS is one of the most common conditions that create a challenge for the RV. Although the mechanism is not completely understood, the hypothesis is based on pathophysiologic changes in the pulmonary vasculature (hyperinflammation based) and the alteration in thoracic pressure (positive pressure ventilation based).

Pulmonary vascular dysfunction in patients with ARDS has been described in the 1977 ground breaking study by Zapol and Snider.[14] These researchers evaluated mechanically ventilated patients who progressively presented with elevated pulmonary vascular resistance and increasingly elevated RV stroke-work index leading to progressive RV dysfunction. In these cases inducing pulmonary dysfunction included a complex myriad of cofactors contributing to the acute progression of ACP. Some of the proposed causes are listed in **Table 2**.

The pulmonary vasculature responds at a local level to the absence of alveolar oxygen by constricting the capillary beds surrounding the sacs, effectively shifting the blood flow to more functional alveoli. This places a resistance load on the fairly ineffective RV; that is, the pulmonary bed is normally very distensible with slight resistance, requiring little RV tension or work to encourage ejection. Because this process in shock is acute, the RV does not adapt to the situation, becoming more dilated and less functional. The pulmonary arterial systolic, mean, and diastolic pressures are vital in evaluating this dysfunction. Pulmonary vascular resistance calculations in this scenario become meaningless. RV support may be critical at this time.

As the septal wall shifts from the overworked RV toward the LV, pulmonary venous pressures increase. Fluid extravasates into the pulmonary interstitium, widening the distance between the alveolus and capillary (diffusion distance). This process further limits gas exchange and is seen on chest radiograph as edema. In addition, if the patient has an inflammatory state (systemic inflammatory response syndrome or septic shock), the capillary walls are "leaky" allowing the efflux of fluid and particles into the pulmonary interstitium and overwhelming surfactant production and ability to oppose alveolar fluid entry, and the sodium pump mechanism, which keeps the alveoli dry. The inflammation of the lung is close behind, destroying the delicate alveolar surfaces and promoting acute respiratory distress (ARDS).

Although the destruction of alveolar walls is considered irreparable, the concomitant alveolar collapse, edema formation, and reduction in pulmonary blood flow are manipulated with mechanical or circuit PEEP strategies and aggressive mobility. To achieve distended alveoli, air trapping on expiration is promoted. Because positive pressure on inspiration is part of ventilator support, the drop of the pressure on expiration reverses the suction pump phenomena; that is, the patient has a significant reduction in filling during inspiration, and primary, limited filling takes place on expiration. The

Table 2 Clues and cues of right heart failure	
Elevated right-sided filling pressures	CVP >12 mm Hg
Right-sided third heart sound	S3 or S4 heard louder during inspiration
Tricuspid regurgitation	Blowing murmur between S1 and S2 heard louder on inspiration
Pulsatile liver	—
Positive hepatojugular reflex	Compression of liver for 20 s distends the neck veins

addition of expiratory positive pressures (PEEP, inverse ratio, rate >20, jet, oscillation) further limits filling. The very strategies used to promote gas exchange may limit the compliance, and therefore filling of both the left and right heart and absolutely places a greater workload on the RV.[15]

The more positive pressure applied in both inspiratory and expiratory cycles, the further limited ventricular filling becomes, as the positive intrathoracic pressure communicates across the myocardium and effectively tamponades the heart. The RA and PCW pressures continue to rise and equalize, the pulmonary artery pressures increase, systemic pressures decrease, urine output drops, systemic and pulmonary edema worsen, and the patient gains fluid weight as volume engorges the veins (**Fig. 7**).

It is hoped that intracardiac pressure monitoring provides a method for the measurement of volume, but because it is also profoundly affected by the compliance of the ventricle, alterations in pulmonary vascular compliance, and ventilator management, these pressures may not be a reliable indicator of true volume load. The other traditional indicators for adequate volume resuscitation, such as blood pressure, heart rate, and urine outputs, are also unreliable as indicative parameters.

KEY CONCEPTS

Ventricular function is not solely about the pressure measures of filling (CVP or RA pressure for RV and pulmonary arterial occlusion pressure [PaOP] or pulmonary artery diastolic pressure [PAD] for LV). When volume is administered or positive pressure is applied it is possible that

1. The RV dilates and becomes noncompliant
2. The septal wall shifts and the LV is compressed (septal shift) and becomes noncompliant

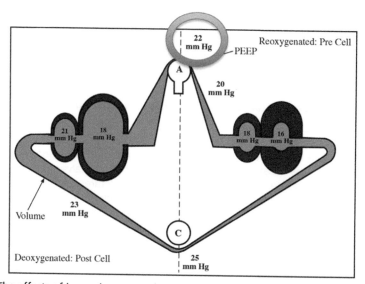

Fig. 7. The effects of increasing mean airway pressure strategies (eg, high PEEP, prolonged inspiratory time, airway pressure release ventilation, and bi-level).

3. Filling of the LV is decreased and affected by intrathoracic pressure changes
4. Tissue delivery of oxygen is decreased
5. Compensatory increase in heart rate occurs, shortening filling time and increasing filling pressure
6. The filling veins engorge
7. Interstitial edema forms
8. Oxygen diffuses less into blood from alveoli

Application of Positive Pressure Ventilation

1. Circuit or mechanical PEEP increases intrapleural pressure and intracardiac pressure, and decreases compliance
2. Circuit or mechanical PEEP increases RV afterload, which in the acute situation profoundly affects the architecture of the RV
3. Positive pressure on inspiration and expiration limits the thoracic pump
4. The RV dilates, because it cannot acutely hypertrophy
5. The PA is engorged with volume

LV dysfunction may not be the most important parameter in this patient population. One of the main assumptions underlying PA catheter interpretation is that changes primarily reflect LV function, despite the undisputed fact that the PA catheter is a right heart catheter. The measured information is profoundly influenced by changes to the compliance of the right heart (preload), the intrathoracic pressures, and the compliance of the pulmonary vasculature (RV afterload). Injurious mechanical ventilation with high inspiratory pressure and large tidal volumes may worsen pulmonary vascular dysfunction inducing pulmonary hypertension and RV dysfunction. The incidence of acute RV failure is around 25% with lung-protective ventilation, and may be much higher depending on the severity of lung injury and the chosen ventilator strategy.[16,17] RV dysfunction has been validated in 25% of patients in multiple clinical trials.

Electrocardiogram signs of RV dysfunction are varied and inconsistent. Signs and symptoms, although not specific to ACP, may generate the decision to follow the patient with echocardiogram (see **Table 2**).

An acute ACP or RV dysfunction is presented as RV dilation. The size of the RV is compared with the LV diameter. A proportional ratio greater than 0.6 indicates RV dysfunction, whereas a ratio of greater than 1.0 indicates severe RV dysfunction.[18–20]

The Relationship between Left Ventricular Outflow and Arterial Perfusion Is Dynamic and Interactive

Traditional cardiac output/cardiac index are measured directly in the pulmonary artery; however, like PCW, these measures indirectly reflect LV function (ejection and filling). Because these measurements are evaluated in the prealveolar compartment, they are subtly or aggressively influenced by the structures at the A-C interface (**Fig. 7**). In a patient in shock, it may be essential to consider the effects of ventilation, pulmonary parenchymal changes, and hypoxemia and volume load when interpreting the measured parameters. Two common and inexpensive methods for validating LV outflow are available in all centers: the monitoring of mean arterial pressure and base deficit or serum bicarbonate, and anion gap.

The relationship of arterial pressure and blood flow dynamics is often a misleading one. As blood flow decreases, either because of loss of ventricular substance, decreased LV volume, or vascular tone changes, the compensatory mechanism is created by sympathetic nervous system discharge. The arterioles and venules constrict to maximize the driving perfusion pressure (mean arterial pressure) and increase volume return to the right heart via an increase in the pressure gradient. In this case, blood pressure becomes profoundly affected by the vasoconstriction and less indicative of blood flow. When auscultating or automatically measuring the blood pressure, the sounds of arterial wall rebounding as blood flows under the occlusive cuff may reflect a number that is misleading. When compared with invasive arterial pressure, the noninvasive measures may be much higher. The key is to follow the mean pressure on both, and to only validate invasive pressure with frequency resonance testing.

Systemic vascular resistance is a derived parameter that reflects a fractionated equation of the resistance circuit divided by the cardiac output or cardiac index. Validation of LV outflow must be performed not in the pulmonary arterial bed, but at the tissue with perfusion indicators. An indicator of adequate tissue perfusion, base excess (deficit), is commonly found on the arterial blood gas. The base varies in direct proportion to the levels of tissue acid, which increase in abnormal metabolic states, such as renal failure, ketosis, and tissue hypoxia or anoxia.

KEY CONCEPTS

In the critical patient, end points should include (1) base measures (-2 to $+2$); (2) lactic acid trends; (3) mean arterial pressure, rather than systemic vascular resistance (reflecting the cardiac index or cardiac output as the denominator) or diastolic pressure (more reflective of vascular tone); and (4) stroke volume and stroke volume indices measured in the systemic arteries.

The patient in acute shock may present with misleading direct and derived information measured at the bedside. Evaluation of hemodynamic data must always be performed with a correlation of tissue acidosis. As inflammation/shock (hypermetabolism) persists, the patient may develop an oxygen extraction deficit, heralded by a base deficit, organ indicators of dysfunction; and as an oxygen extraction deficit persists the patient may develop subsequent myocardial dysfunction, delivery failure, organ failure, and profound acidosis.

SUMMARY

In caring for the acutely ill patients with heart failure, the provider must make a distinct effort to evaluate the oxyhemodynamic profile with certain points in mind.

- The RV does not acutely adjust to an increase in work
- The RV dilates, because it cannot acutely hypertrophy
- As the RV dilates and becomes noncompliant, the LV is compressed and becomes noncompliant
- The filling veins engorge
- Interstitial edema forms
- The patient has relative arterial hypovolemia
- Tissue extraction of oxygen is decreased, and a compensatory increase in heart rate occurs, further decreasing filling
- Pulmonary blood flow past the alveoli is limited
- The patient exhibits signs of refractory hypoxemia with a wide $AaDo_2$ and a low P/F ratio, and the tissues and organs express a hypoxic or anoxic state

The dynamics of these patients may be misleading because they present with refractory hypotension, weight gain, and decreasing urine output. Echocardiographic

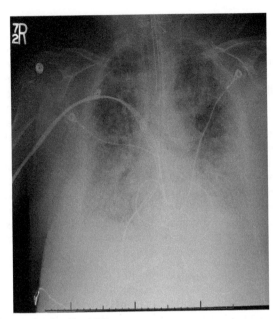

Fig. 8. Chest radiograph of patient T.S.

analysis, pulmonary arterial pressure monitoring, and RA/RV pressures should be evaluated and may be reflective of ventilator management pulmonary manipulation and affected by the additional affects of RV dysfunction.

SIMPLE STRATEGIES

For patients with diagnosed RV dysfunction and ARDS, echocardiogram needs to be used to evaluate the effects of positive pressure on the RF performance and LV filling. Evaluating the effects of ventilation changes on the RV limits tidal volume and application of PEEP, while avoiding the effects of hypercapnia-induced pulmonary

Table 3
The arterial blood gas analysis over the first 4 hours of patient T.S.

Time/Date/Measure	2/22 0115 Arterial	2/22 0527 Arterial	2/22 Venous	2/22 0818 Arterial
pH	7.31	7.48	7.35	7.31
Po_2	88	98	30	95
Pco_2	21	21	37	58
Base deficit	13.9	6.7	5.3	8.0
Sao_2	90%	95%	—	92%
Svo_2	—	—	40%	—
FiO_2	1.0	0.8	—	0.6
PEEP	8	15	—	17
CVP	—	14	—	24

Abbreviation: FiO_2, fraction of inspired oxygen.

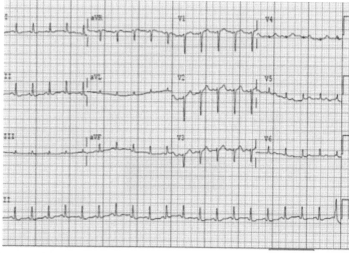

Fig. 9. Electrocardiogram of patient T.S.

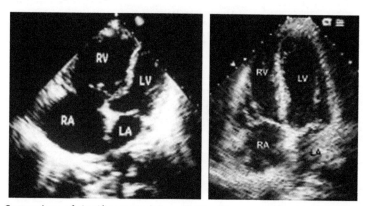

Fig. 10. Comparison of significant RV failure (*left*) with normal diameter (*right*).

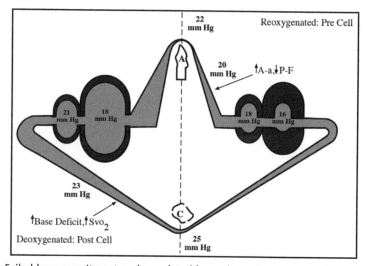

Fig. 11. Failed lung recruitment and correlated hemodynamic parameters in patient T.S.

A

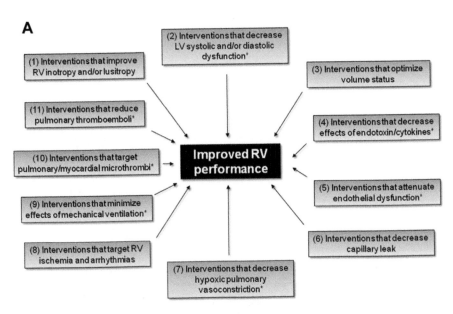

(2) Interventions that decrease LV systolic and/or diastolic dysfunction*

(1) Interventions that improve RV inotropy and/or lusitropy

(3) Interventions that optimize volume status

(11) Interventions that reduce pulmonary thromboemboli*

(4) Interventions that decrease effects of endotoxin/cytokines*

(10) Interventions that target pulmonary/myocardial microthrombi*

Improved RV performance

(5) Interventions that attenuate endothelial dysfunction*

(9) Interventions that minimize effects of mechanical ventilation*

(8) Interventions that target RV ischemia and arrhythmias

(6) Interventions that decrease capillary leak

(7) Interventions that decrease hypoxic pulmonary vasoconstriction*

B

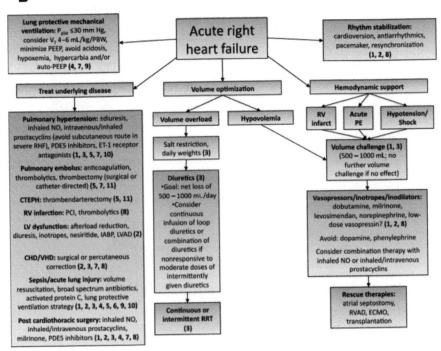

Lung protective mechanical ventilation: P_{plat} ≤30 mm Hg, consider V_t 4–6 mL/kg/PBW, minimize PEEP, avoid acidosis, hypoxemia, hypercarbia and/or auto-PEEP **(4, 7, 9)**

Acute right heart failure

Rhythm stabilization: cardioversion, antiarrhythmics, pacemaker, resynchronization **(1, 2, 8)**

Treat underlying disease

Volume optimization

Hemodynamic support

Pulmonary hypertension: ±diuresis, inhaled NO, intravenous/inhaled prostacyclins (avoid subcutaneous route in severe RHF), PDE5 inhibitors, ET-1 receptor antagonists **(1, 3, 5, 7, 10)**

Pulmonary embolus: anticoagulation, thrombolytics, thrombectomy (surgical or catheter-directed) **(5, 7, 11)**

CTEPH: thrombendarterectomy **(5, 11)**

RV infarction: PCI, thrombolytics **(8)**

LV dysfunction: afterload reduction, diuresis, inotropes, nesiritide, IABP, LVAD **(2)**

CHD/VHD: surgical or percutaneous correction **(2, 3, 7, 8)**

Sepsis/acute lung injury: volume resuscitation, broad spectrum antibiotics, activated protein C, lung protective ventilation strategy **(1, 2, 3, 4, 5, 6, 9, 10)**

Post cardiothoracic surgery: inhaled NO, inhaled/intravenous prostacyclins, milrinone, PDE5 inhibitors **(1, 2, 3, 4, 7, 8)**

Volume overload

Hypovolemia

RV infarct

Acute PE

Hypotension/Shock

Salt restriction, daily weights **(3)**

Volume challenge **(1, 3)** (500 – 1000 mL; no further volume challenge if no effect)

Diuretics **(3)**
•Goal: net loss of 500 – 1000 mL/day
•Consider continuous infusion of loop diuretics or combination of diuretics if nonresponsive to moderate doses of intermittently given diuretics

Vasopressors/inotropes/inodilators: dobutamine, milrinone, levosimendan, norepinephrine, low-dose vasopressin? **(1, 2, 8)**

Avoid: dopamine, phenylephrine

Consider combination therapy with inhaled NO or inhaled/intravenous prostacyclins

Continuous or intermittent RRT **(3)**

Rescue therapies: atrial septostomy, RVAD, ECMO, transplantation

vasoconstriction. When circulation is impaired in RV dysfunction, limiting mean airway pressure and fluid resuscitation may be important. Reducing volume through diuresis and ultrafiltration may yield favorable results, as may consideration of RV inotropic support and pulmonary vasodilation (**Fig. 8**).

CASE PRESENTATION

T.S. is a 64-year-old woman with an antithrombin III deficiency on warfarin with history of multiple pulmonary emboli status post inferior vena-caval filter, chronic pancreatitis, metastasis, osteoporosis, and chronic pain disorder who presents with AMS and acute respiratory failure. The patient has had 3 days of a wet cough with hemoptysis of bright red blood and clots associated with chest pain, increased difficulty breathing, and chills. Three days before admission she also had new-onset left, lower extremity weakness and numbness that interfere with walking. She has fallen three times in the last 2 days before admission, and 4 hours ago fell, hit the back of her head, could not get up, and became increasingly unresponsive. Emergency medical services were called. On presentation to the emergency department her SpO_2 was 40% but improved to 80% when on a nonrebreather. She was emergently intubated for respiratory failure and received a 4 L bolus of 0.9% sodium chloride. Her admission laboratory analysis showed a total white blood count of 19.4 and total serum CO_2 of 18 mEq indicating metabolic acidosis; the arterial blood gas analysis over the first 4 hours is shown in **Table 3**.

Chest radiograph exposed significant ARDS (see **Fig. 8**) and the electrocardiogram was relatively normal (**Fig. 9**). However, after intubation and application of invasive ventilation via synchronized intermittent mandatory ventilation (SIMV) with low tidal volume ventilation, hypoxia was treated with a rapid increase in PEEP, resulting in significant hypoperfusion, acidosis, increasing CVP, and decreasing urine output. Within 24 hours the patient became febrile to 103°F, blood pressure of 84/54, heart rate of 145, respiratory rate of 41. Shock was clinically apparent. The echocardiogram (**Fig. 10**) revealed RV dysfunction (**Figs. 11** and **12**). Pulmonary embolus was ruled out and all attempts were made to support the right heart and decrease the PEEP. Despite the implementation of maximized vasopressors, inotropes, pulmonary vasodilation, and prone position, T.S. succumbed to her overwhelming sepsis and acute right heart failure.

Fig. 12. (*A*) Categorization of therapeutic interventions aimed at improving RV function in the intensive care unit interventions marked with an *asterisk* directly or indirectly decrease right ventricular (RV) afterload. (*B*) Treatment of acute right ventricular failure in the intensive care unit. Numbers in parentheses refer to the treatment categories outlined in Fig. 12A. In addition to the strategies depicted in the figure, general measures, such as oxygen administration, nutritional support, and prophylactic measures, should be applied. CHD/VHD, congenital/valvular heart disease; CTEPH, chronic thromboembolic pulmonary hypertension; ECMO, extracorporeal membrane oxygenation; ET-1, endothelin-1; IABP, intra-aortic balloon pump; LVAD/RVAD, left/right ventricular assist device; NO, nitric oxide; PBW, predicted body weight; PCI, percutaneous coronary intervention; PDE5, phosphodiesterase 5; PE, pulmonary embolism; Pplat, plateau pressure; RRT, renal replacement therapy; VT, tidal volume. (*From* Lahm T, McCaslin CA, Wozniak TC, et al. Medical and surgical treatment of acute right ventricular failure. J Am Coll Cardiol 2010;56(18):1441; with permission.)

REFERENCES

1. Vieillard-Baron A, Loubieres Y, Schmitt JM, et al. Cyclic changes in right ventricular output impedance during mechanical ventilation. J Appl Physiol 1999;87(5): 1644–50.
2. Guervilly C, Forel JM, Hraiech S, et al. Right ventricular function during high-frequency oscillatory ventilation in adults with acute respiratory distress syndrome. Crit Care Med 2012;40(5):1539–45.
3. Vieillard-Baron A, Prin S, Chergui K, et al. Echo-Doppler demonstration of acute cor pulmonale at the bedside in the medical intensive care unit. Am J Respir Crit Care Med 2002;166(10):1310–9.
4. Pinsky MR, Desmet JM, Vincent JL. Effect of positive end expiratory pressure on right ventricular function in humans. Am Rev Respir Dis 1992;146(3):681–7.
5. Vieillard-Baron A, Price L, Matthay M. Acute cor pulmonale in ARDS. Intensive Care Med 2013;39(10):1836–8.
6. Vieillard-Baron A, Jardin F. Acute right ventricular dysfunction: focus on acute cor pulmonale. In: Hill NS, Farber HW, editors. Pulmonary Hypertension. New York: Humana Press; 2008.
7. Cheatham ML, Nelson LD, Chang MC, et al. Right ventricular end-diastolic volume index as a predictor of preload status in-patients on positive end-expiratory pressure. Crit Care Med 1998;26(11):1801–6.
8. Repessé X, Charron C, Vieillard-Baron A. Acute cor pulmonale in ARDS. Chest 2015;147(1):259–65.
9. Zapol WM, Kobayashi K, Snider MT, et al. Vascular obstruction causes pulmonary hypertension in severe acute respiratory failure. Chest 1977;71(Suppl 2):306–7.
10. Jardin F, Dubourg O, Bourdarias JP. Echocardiographic pattern of acute cor pulmonale. Chest 1997;111(1):209–17.
11. Kirton OC, Civetta JM. Do pulmonary artery catheters alter outcome in trauma patients? New Horizons 1997;5(3):222–7.
12. Chang MC, Mondy JS, Meredith JW, et al. Clinical application of ventricular end-systolic elastance and the ventricular pressure-volume diagram. Shock 1997; 7(6):413–9.
13. Reichert CL, Visser CA, van den Brink RB, et al. Prognostic value of biventricular function in hypotensive patients after cardiac surgery as assessed by transesophageal echocardiography. J Cardiothorac Vasc Anesth 1992;6(4): 429–32.
14. Zapol WM, Snider MT. Pulmonary hypertension in severe acute respiratory failure. N Engl J Med 1977;296(9):476–80.
15. Lansdorp B, Hofhuizen C, Lavieren M, et al. Mechanical ventilation induced intrathoracic pressure distribution and heart-lung interactions. Crit Care Med 2014;42: 1983–90.
16. Boissier F, Katsahian S, Razazi K, et al. Prevalence and prognosis of cor pulmonale during protective ventilation for acute respiratory distress syndrome. Intensive Care Med 2013;39(10):1725–33.
17. Chiumello D, Pesenti A. The monitoring of acute cor pulmonale is still necessary in "Berlin" ARDS patients. Intensive Care Med 2013;39(10):1864–6.
18. Rudski LG, Lai WW, Afi lalo J, et al. Guidelines for the echocardiographic assessment of the right heart in adults: a report from the American Society of Echocardiography endorsed by the European Association of Echocardiography, a registered branch of the European Society of Cardiology, and the Canadian Society of Echocardiography. J Am Soc Echocardiogr 2010;23(7):685–713.

19. Ryan T, Petrovic O, Dillon JC, et al. An echocardiographic index for separation of right ventricular volume and pressure overload. J Am Coll Cardiol 1985;5(4): 918–27.
20. Huh J, Koh Y. Ventilation parameters used to guide cardiopulmonary function during mechanical ventilation. Curr Opin Crit Care 2013;19(3):215–20.

Mechanisms of Cardiotoxicity and the Development of Heart Failure

 CrossMark

Christopher S. Lee, PhD, RN

KEYWORDS

- Cardiotoxicity • Heart failure • Pathophysiology • Cardiomyopathy • Toxicity

KEY POINTS

- The term, *cardiotoxicity*, generally refers to toxicity of a substance that negatively affects the heart but also has been described using more precise clinical terms in cancer trials.
- Common mechanisms of cardiotoxicity associated with cancer therapies include direct cardiomyocyte injury, thromboembolic events, and hypertension.
- Anti–tumor necrosis factor (TNF)-α agents used in the treatment of rheumatoid arthritis may interfere with ischemic preconditioning or other roles of low levels of inflammation in cell repair.
- Alcohol results in cardiotoxicity via oxidative stress, apoptosis, mitochondrial stress, and protein catabolism.
- Cocaine is cardiotoxic primarily by means of sympathetic nervous system stimulation of heart and smooth muscle cells.

INTRODUCTION

Despite its inherent resiliency and redundant physiologic mechanisms that foster rhythmic muscular contraction, the heart is vulnerable to both naturally occurring and synthetic toxins. Cardiotoxicity (ie, toxicity that negatively affects the heart)[1] can play an important role in both the development and worsening of cardiovascular disease in general and in heart failure (HF) in particular.[2] HF is the fastest growing cardiovascular disorder and the primary reason for hospitalization among older adults.[3–6] Thus, knowledge about medicines and other substances that impair the mechanical and/or electronic functions of the heart is important to providing care for patients who are at risk for or who have already developed the quality and duration of life

Disclosure statement: The author has nothing to disclose.
School of Nursing and Knight Cardiovascular Institute, Oregon Health and Science University, Mail Code: SN-2N, 3455 SW, US Veterans Hospital Road, Portland, OR 97239-2941, USA
E-mail address: leechri@ohsu.edu

limiting condition of HF.[7–11] Accordingly, the purpose of this article is to synthesize what is known about common mechanisms of cardiotoxicity and how they relate to the development of HF.

There are several drugs used in the treatment of extracardiovascular diseases that are known to contribute to the development of left ventricular dysfunction and/or the clinical syndrome of HF. For example, several cancer therapies and biologic agents used in the management of chronic inflammatory conditions like rheumatoid arthritis are well-known for their cardiotoxic effects. Additionally, long-term use of alcohol and cocaine are also known contributors to the development of cardiomyopathy and the syndrome of HF.

CANCER THERAPIES AND CARDIOTOXICITY

Comorbidities after cancer and cancer therapies are a growing public health concern. Ccardiovascular disease is now a competing cause of morbidity and mortality among cancer survivors,[12–15] making surveillance for conditions like HF equally if not more important to cancer surveillance.[16] A vast majority of the world's literature on cardiotoxicity focuses on agents used in the treatment of cancer, including chemotherapies and targeted therapies. Although there is no consensus regarding a clinical interpretation of toxicity that negatively affects the heart, the cardiac review and evaluation committee for trials involving the drug trastuzumab (Herceptin) defined cardiotoxicity in a way that is tangible to most clinicians (**Table 1**).[17] In brief, cardiotoxicity typically refers to cardiomyopathy, signs and symptoms of HF, or clinically significant reductions in left ventricular ejection fraction. Each class, specific agent, and combination of therapies used in the treatment of various cancers comes with differential risks for the development of HF[18] and vary in mechanisms of cardiotoxicity. The many nuances of cardiotoxicity associated with specific cancer therapies are reviewed in detail elsewhere[19,20] and are beyond the scope of this article. In general, however, cardiotoxicity in response to cancer therapies can result from direct cardiomyocyte injury or inflammation, thromboembolic events and subsequent ischemia, and/or therapy-induced hypertension.[20]

Direct Cardiomyocyte Injury

Common mechanisms of direct cardiomyocyte injury associated with cancer therapies include myofibril disarray that leads to poor contractility, reactive oxygen species (ROS) formation that leads to oxidative stress and cell injury/death, and mitochondrial

Table 1 Trastuzumab trials cardiac review and evaluation committee criteria for cardiotoxicity	
1	Cardiomyopathy characterized by a decrease in left ventricular ejection fraction that is either global or more severe in the septum.
2	Symptoms of congestive heart failure.
3	Signs of heart failure, including but not limited to S3 gallop, tachycardia, or both.
4	Decline in left ventricular ejection fraction of a. ≥5% To below 55% with accompanying signs or symptoms of heart failure, or b. ≥10% To below 55% without accompanying signs or symptoms.

Note: Any 1 of the 4 criteria was sufficient to confirm a diagnosis of cardiac dysfunction.
Adapted from Seidman A, Hudis C, Pierri MK, et al. Cardiac dysfunction in the trastuzumab clinical trials experience. J Clin Oncol 2002;20(5):1215–21.

dysfunction that impairs most actions of cardiomyocytes (**Fig. 1**). For example, anthracyclines that are a mainstay of breast cancer treatment give rise to myofibrilar disarray and subsequent poor contractility.[21,22] Specifically, anthracyclines induce degradation of critical components of the sarcomere, like titin, by calcium-dependent kinases, like calpain.[23,24] Anthracyclines prolong the opening time of calcium channels on the

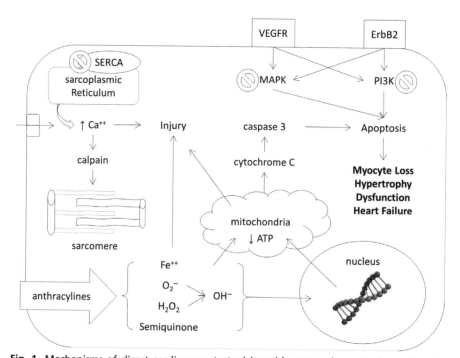

Fig. 1. Mechanisms of direct cardiomyocyte toxicity with cancer drugs. Anthracyclines increase intracellular calcium by several means, including prolonging the opening time of ion channels, such as the ryanodine channel on the sarcoplasmic reticulum, and L-type calcium channels on the cell membrane, and inhibiting the reuptake of calcium through the sarcoplasmic reticulum ATPase. Increased intracellular calcium stimulates calpain to break down critical components of the sarcomere, like titin, and also results in the expression of noncontractile proteins and fibrosis. In addition to calcium toxicity, another common mechanism of cardiotoxicity is oxidative stress. Anthracyclines, as an example, enter cardiomyocytes via passive diffusion and give rise to several ROS, including semiquinone, O_2^- and H_2O_2. These ROS can cause direct cell injury and death but also can give rise to free iron and hyper-ROS, like OH^-, that can result in direct damage to DNA and subsequent decrease in mitochondrial ATP production. In response to several cancer drugs, mitochondria release cytochrome C that brings about apoptosis through the actions of caspase 3. Cancer drugs that block VEGF or VEGFRs or downstream intracellular processes thereof alter several cell survival signals within cardiomyocytes, including the MAPK and PI3K pathways; ErbB2 receptors are also associated with the MAPK and PI3K survival pathways. Thus, apoptosis is a common mechanism of cardiotoxicity with cancer drugs that target VEGF or ErbB2 receptors and results in myocyte loss, hypertrophy, ventricular dysfunction, and eventually heart failure. ATP, adenosine triphosphate; Ca^{++}, calcium; ErbB2, ErbB2 (otherwise known as the HER2/neu receptor); Fe^{++}, iron; H_2O_2, hydrogen peroxide; MAPK, mitogen-activated protein kinase; O_2^-, oxide; OH^-, hydroxyl; PI3K, phosphatidylinositide 3-kinase; SERCA, sarcoplasmic reticulum calcium adenosine triphosphatase; VEGF, vascular endothelial growth factor; VEGFR, VEGF receptor.

sarcoplasmic reticulum, enhance the activity of calcium channels on the cell membrane, and inhibit the reuptake of calcium into the sarcoplasmic reticulum, which collectively increase intracellular calcium.[25,26] Increased intracellular calcium is a major driver of cardiotoxicity in response to anthracyclines. Calcium toxicity eventually results in hypertrophy[27] and expression of noncontractile proteins[28] and fibrosis[29] and consequently sets the stage for the development of HF. Anthracyclines also enter cardiomyocytes via passive diffusion and cause the accumulation of ROS, such as semiquinone, oxide, and hydrogen peroxide.[30] These ROS also increase intracellular free iron that can lead to direct damage to DNA and the conversion of oxide and hydrogen peroxide to one of the most potent ROS hydroxyls.[30] Finally, anthracyclines impair the mitochondrial production of adenosine triphosphate[19,30] that is essential for the many cardiomyocyte functions that are energy dependent, like contraction and calcium reuptake.

There are several cancer therapies that target vascular endothelial growth factor (VEGF) and associated receptors. For example, bevacizumab is a monoclonal antibody to VEGF, and there are tyrosine kinase receptor inhibitors that target VEGF receptors, such as sunitinib and sorafenib.[25] Although the targets of such therapies are tumor cells, these receptors are also expressed on cardiomyocytes. Under normal physiologic conditions, VEGF is cardioprotective.[19] By inhibiting VEGF, VEGF receptors, or VEGF intracellular signaling, several cancer therapies can result in cardiotoxicity via impairing cardiomyocyte survival signaling (see **Fig. 1**).[25,30] The targets of other cancer therapies are expressed on cardiomyocytes in addition to the target cancer cells. For example, ErbB2 – the target of trastuzumab – is expressed on cardiomyocytes. ErbB2 receptors are essential for normal cardiomyocyte function; that is, the cell signaling pathways associated with ErbB2 typically promote cell survival.[24] Cardiotoxicity associated with trastuzumab is thought to be associated with (1) hypertrophic response to altered ErbB2 signaling,[19] (2) adenoside triphosphate depletion,[31] and (3) increased susceptibility to anthracyclines that are frequently administered together with trastuzumab.[20] A potential cardiotoxic mechanism of the taxane pactitaxel is the release of histamine that may result in conduction disturbances.[20]

Thromboembolic Events

Arterial thromboembolism can result from broad-spectrum angiogenesis inhibitors like thalidomide and lenalidomide.[20] Although the exact mechanism of thromboembolism in response to these agents is unclear, disruption of the integrity of the vascular endothelium and subsequent platelet activation has been proposed.[32] Venous thromboembolism can result from antineoplastic agents. For example, cisplatin use is associated with platelet aggregation, prothrombotic lipid formation (eg, thromboxane), and arachidonic acid pathway activation[33] that can collectively result in thromboembolism. Other substances, such as anthracyclines, potentially disrupt vascular endothelial function by targeting adherens junctions between cells.[34] Thromboembolism within coronary arteries can result in tissue injury and/or infarction and set the stage for the development of HF.

Hypertension

Hypertension is a common antecedent to the development of HF and a common adverse cardiovascular consequence of cancer treatment. Hypertension is most commonly seen with VEGF inhibitors.[35] Under normal physiologic conditions, VEGF increases synthesis of the vasodilator nitric oxide through up-regulation of endothelial nitric oxide synthase.[36] Consequently, a likely hypertensive mechanism of VEGF inhibitors involves decreased nitric oxide synthase production that reduces the production of nitric oxide (**Fig. 2**). A decrease in nitric oxide availability leads to constriction of vascular smooth muscles and subsequent increases in blood pressure.[37] The cardiotoxicity of 5-fluorouracil also is mediated through the drug's influence on the vascular endothelia, including decreased production of endothelial nitric oxide synthase that can cause vasoconstriction. The pressure overload associated with high blood pressure is a major risk factor for the development of HF.

BIOLOGICAL AGENTS AND HEART FAILURE

There are several commercially available biological agents used in the treatment of rheumatoid arthritis that are associated with the development and/or worsening of HF. The specific cardiovascular effects of specific rheumatoid arthritis therapies are reviewed in detail elsewhere.[38] Several pathogenic processes of rheumatoid arthritis are associated with the development of HF, such as vasculitis, arrhythmias, valve disease, pericarditis, and cardiomyopathy, that are independent of treatment with biological agents.[39] Drugs that influence TNF-α are of most interest in the development of HF. TNF-α originates from activated macrophages,[40] monocytes, T cells and B cells,[41] and cardiomyocytes.[42] The biggest concern with high levels of TNF-α in HF is their negative inotropic effects.[40] Low levels of TNF-α, however, may be cardioprotective in response to acute ischemia through protective preconditioning and may play an important role in cell repair.[43] Low levels of TNF-α also may stimulate nitric oxide production in endothelial cells and help protect adjacent cardiomyocytes from mechanical stress.[44] Monoclonal antibodies to TNF-α were developed to ameliorate the negative inotropic and pro-remodeling effects of high levels of TNF-α in HF, but these drugs were not efficacious,[45,46] perhaps for the reasons outlined previously. Similarly, the anti–TNF-α therapies used in the treatment of rheumatoid arthritis may block the cardioprotective effects of low levels of TNF-α,[43] possibly explaining why these therapies may induce HF,[47,48] and also explain the lack of efficacy of anti–TNF-α agents in patients with advanced HF.[49] Because of a lack of consensus and sufficient data, it is currently recommended that patients with class I or II HF treated with anti-TNFα agents be monitored for the worsening of HF and that patients with class III or IV HF not be treated with anti–TNF-α agents.[44]

ALCOHOLIC CARDIOMYOPATHY

Long-term and heavy alcohol use is associated with the development of dilated cardiomyopathy.[50] The pathogenesis of alcoholic cardiomyopathy is complex, but several dominant mechanisms have been proposed, including oxidative stress, apoptosis, mitochondrial stress, alterations in metabolism, and protein catabolism.[51] The metabolism of ethanol can directly result in oxidative stress within cardiomyocytes by means of synthesis of several ROS and decreased synthesis of antioxidants (**Fig. 3**). Additionally, increase in the intercellular actions of catecholamines, like norepinephrine and angiotensin II, that are known to be elevated in alcoholic cardiomyopathy also give rise to the synthesis of several ROS and also cause cellular apoptosis. The key cellular consequences of alcohol on cardiomyocytes are oxidative stress, apoptosis, mitochondrial dysfunction, increased intracellular calcium accompanied by decreased calcium sensitivity, contractile protein dysfunction, and the reduced synthesis and accelerated degradation of contractile and other critical proteins. The cumulative influence of these cellular mechanisms over time are impaired muscle contraction and relaxation, decreased cardiac output and increased preload, chamber dilation, and wall thinning accompanied by hypertrophy of normal cells.

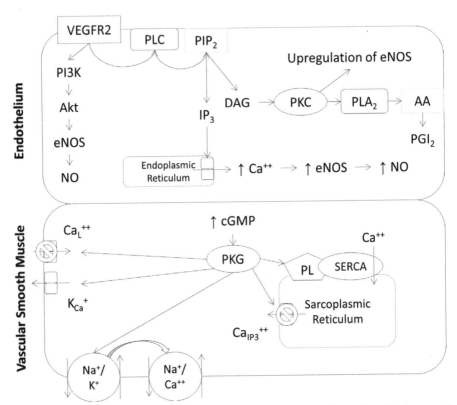

Fig. 2. VEGF and vasodilatation. NO production induced by VEGF is mediated by increased intracellular Ca^{++}. The VEGF receptor (VEGFR2) increases the activity of PLC, which in turn hydrolyzes PIP_2 into IP_3 and DAG. IP_3 activates IP_3-gated calcium channels on the endoplasmic reticulum and causes increased intercellular Ca^{++}, which is a major driver of eNOS and eventual NO production. DAG leads to activation of PKC and PLA_2 that released AA from membrane lipids and generates PGI_2. VEGFR activity is also involved with the PI3K pathway that includes activation of Akt-phosphorylation of eNOS and providing a mechanism for NO synthesis that is not dependent on Ca^{++}. NO and PGI_2 promote vasodilatation in adjacent vascular smooth muscle cells by increase cGMP. cGMP stimulates PKG, which leads to vasodilatation via 4 main mechanisms. First, PKG phosphorylates Ca_L^{++} and causes membrane hyperpolarization by activating K_{Ca}^+; thus, there is less intracellular calcium for contraction and the cells become less responsive to other mediators of constriction. Second, PKG accelerates sodium/potassium pumps, which in turn fuels greater sodium/calcium exchange and thereby calcium efflux from the intracellular space. Third, PKG inhibits of Ca_{IP3}^{++}, further decreasing intracellular calcium. Finally, PKG phosphorylation of PL accelerates the SERCA and calcium resequestration into the sarcoplasmic reticulum. These actions favor vasodilatation and are disrupted by cancer drugs that influence VEGF. AA, arachadonic acid; Ca^{++}, calcium; Ca_{IP3}^{++}, inositol triphosphate-gated calcium channel; Ca_L^{++}, L-type calcium channel; cGMP, cyclic guanosine monophosphate; DAG, diacylglycerol; eNOS, endothelial NO synthase; IP_3, inositol triphosphate; K_{Ca}^+, calcium-dependent potassium channel; Na^+/Ca^{++}, sodium-calcium exchange; Na^+/K^+, sodium-potassium-ATPase; NO, nitric oxide; PGI_2, prostacyclin; PI3K, phosphatidylinositide 3-kinase; PIP_2, phosphatidylinositol biphosphate; PKC, protein kinase C; PKG, protein kinase G; PL, phospholamban; PLA_2, phospholipase A2; PLC, phospholipase C; SERCA, sarcoplasmic reticulum calcium adenosine triphosphatase.

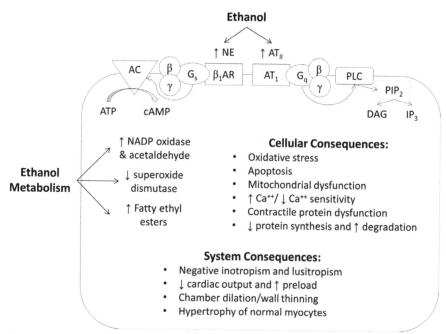

Fig. 3. Influence of ethanol on the heart. Long-term and heavy ethanol use increases both NE and AT_{II}. When NE binds with a β_1AR, the α subunit of the stimulatory G protein dissociates and increases the activity of the enzyme AC. AC generates cAMP from ATP. cAMP acts within cells as the second messenger of NE. When AT_{II} binds with an AT_1, the q subunit dissociates from the G-protein complex and activates PLC. PLC in turn hydrolyzes PIP_2 into IP_3 and DAG that act as the second messengers of AT_{II}. Metabolism of elthanol results in several ROS, including NADP oxidase and acetaldehyde and reduces the production of antioxidants like superoxide dismutase. The metabolism of ethanol also results in the accumulation of fatty ethyl esters within cardiomyocytes. Cumulatively, the actions of the intracellular second messengers of NE and AT_{II} (indirect effects) and the end-products of ethanol metabolism (direct effects) result in a cascade of cellular and system consequences that lead to the development of heart failure. AC, adenylyl cyclase; AT_1, angiotensin II type 1 receptor; AT_{II}, angiotensin II; ATP, adenosine triphosphate; Ca^{++}, calcium; cAMP, cyclic adenosine monophosphate; DAG, diacylglycerol; Gq, Gq protein; Gs, α subunit of the stimulatory G protein; IP_3, inositol triphosphate; NADP, nicotinamide adenine dinucleotide phosphate; NE, norepinephrine; PIP_2, phosphatidylinositol biphosphate; PLC, phospholipase C; β, β subunit of the G protein; β_1AR, $\beta1$-adrenergic receptor; γ, γ subunit of the G protein.

Consequently, long-term heavy alcohol use can lead to the development of the clinical syndrome of HF.

COCAINE AND THE DEVELOPMENT OF HEART FAILURE

Cocaine directly inhibits the reuptake of catecholamines at the site of sympathetic nerve terminals. As a result, adrenergic receptors are particularly sensitive to endogenous norepinephrine in response to cocaine use in both the heart and vascular smooth muscles resulting in increased contractility and elevated blood pressure **(Fig. 4)**.[52] Cocaine also stimulates increased endothelin secretion from endothelial cells that has actions similar to norepinephrine on smooth muscle cells; endothelin, however, is a more potent vasoconstrictor compared with norephinephrine. Via

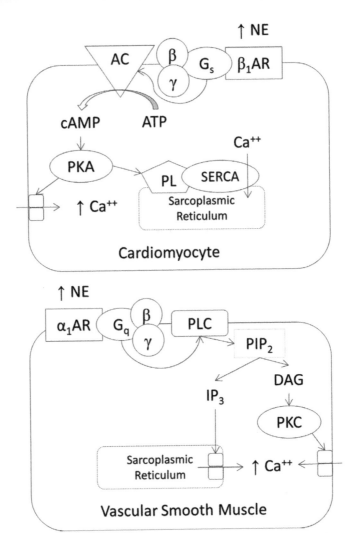

Fig. 4. Contractile and vasoconstrictive effects of cocaine. By blocking reuptake at the site of sympathetic nerve terminals, cocaine results in increased sensitivity to catecholamines like NE. When NE binds with β_1ARs on cardiomyocytes, the α-subunit of the stimulatory G protein dissociates and increases the activity of the enzyme AC. AC generates cAMP from ATP. cAMP activates cAMP-dependent PKA. PKA acts on intracellular protein targets by adding a high-energy phosphate (ie, phosphorylation). Phosphorylation of L-type calcium ion channels increases intracellular Ca^{++} and the force of contraction (ie, positive inotropism). Phosphorylation of PL allows the SERCA to augment the rate of Ca^{++} removal from the intracellular and results in enhanced ventricular relaxation. When NE binds with α_1ARs on vascular smooth muscle cells, the q subunit dissociates from the G-protein complex and activates PLC. PLC in turn hydrolyzes PIP_2 into IP_3 and DAG. IP_3 activates IP_3-gated Ca^{++} channels on the sarcoplasmic reticulum and stimulates enhanced release of Ca^{++} into the intracellular space causing vasoconstriction. DAG stimulates PKC, which in turn phosphorylates Ca^{++} ion channels on the cell membrane and further enhances intracellular Ca^{++}. Collectively, these actions give rise to increased oxygen demand, Ca^{++} toxicity, hypertrophy, and eventually heart failure. AC, adenylyl cyclase; ATP, adenosine triphosphate; Ca^{++}, calcium; cAMP, cyclic adenosine monophosphate; DAG, diacylglycerol; Gq, Gq protein; Gs, α subunit of the stimulatory G protein; IP_3, inositol triphosphate; NE, norepinephrine; PIP_2, phosphatidylinositol biphosphate; PKA, protein kinase A; PKC, protein kinase C; PL, phospholamban; PLC, phospholamban C; SERCA, sarcoplasmic reticulum Ca^{++} adenosine triphosphatase; α_1AR, α-adrenergic receptors; β, β subunit of the G protein; β_1AR, β1-adrenergic receptor; γ, γ subunit of the G protein.

catecholamine reuptake inhibition, cocaine also results in an increase in heart rate by increasing the rate of depolarization of pacemaker cells (**Fig. 5A**). The positive chronotropic, inotropic, and vasoconstrictive properties of cocaine collectively give rise to increased oxygen demand and eventually ischemia and/or infarction and HF. Moreover, vasoconstriction and vasospasm of coronary arteries associated with cocaine can decrease oxygen delivery to the myocardium either directly or as a result of coronary platelet aggregation and/or thrombus formation. Hence, decreased oxygen delivery to myocardial tissue that has increased oxygen demand accelerates tissue ischemia and eventual cardiomyocyte death. Cocaine also has class I antiarrhythmic properties and partially suppresses fast sodium channels as well as potassium channels involved in repolarization (see **Fig. 5B**).[53] Finally, sodium and potassium channel

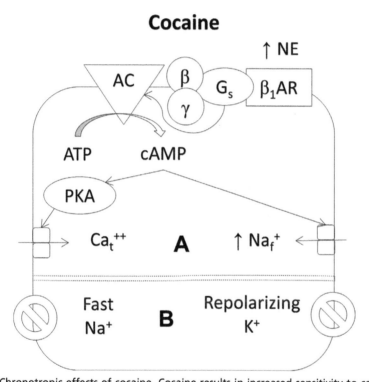

Fig. 5. Chronotropic effects of cocaine. Cocaine results in increased sensitivity to catecholamines like NE. When NE binds with β_1AR on pacemaker cells, the α-subunit of the stimulatory G protein dissociates and increases the activity of the enzyme AC. AC generates cAMP from ATP. cAMP activates PKA. PKA adds a high-energy phosphate to Ca_t^{++} to increases intracellular Ca^{++} during diastolic depolarization (*A*). At the same time, cAMP acts directly on Na_f^+ to increase intracellular sodium during diastolic depolarization. Collectively, the increase in sodium and Ca^{++} accelerate the rate of depolarization of pacemaker cells and with it the heart rate. Cocaine also suppresses fast sodium channels during depolarization and potassium channels involved with repolarization (*B*) altering both the QRS and QT intervals. AC, adenylyl cyclase; ATP, adenosine triphosphate; cAMP, cyclic adenosine monophosphate; Ca^{++}, calcium; Ca_t^{++}, transient calcium ion channels; Gs, α subunit of the stimulatory G protein; K^+, potassium; Na^+, sodium; Na_f^+, funny sodium channels; NE, norepinephrine; PKA, protein kinase A; β, β subunit of the G protein; β_1AR, β1-adrenergic receptor; γ, γ subunit of the G protein.

function with cocaine and the subsequent prolongation of the QRS and QT intervals can give rise to arrhythmias and a further predispose to HF.[53]

SUMMARY

When clinicians think about the natural history of HF, they have a tendency to think about common causes like ischemic heart disease[38,39] and primary hypertension.[37] As reviewed in this article, however, cardiotoxicity plays an important role in the evolution of HF among adults treated for common diseases, like cancer and rheumatoid arthritis, and among those who engage in long-term recreational drug use. In particular, HF should be viewed as a competing cause of morbidity and mortality among cancer survivors given that their risk for cardiovascular disease is greater than cancer remission. There are several pathophysiological mechanisms involved in cardiotoxity, including direct cardiomyocyte injury, thromboembolic events, and hypertension. These and newly emerging mechanisms of cardiotoxicity need to be taken into consideration when considering the risk of developing HF. It is also important to consider that the definition of cardiotoxicity may not capture subclinical pathophysiology that may be missed as part of pharmacovigilance studies. Hence, the definition of cardiotoxicity is likely to advance along with knowledge about how to detect subclinical injury to the myocardium.

REFERENCES

1. Brana I, Tabernero J. Cardiotoxicity. Ann Oncol 2010;21(Suppl 7):vii173-9.
2. Yancy CW, Jessup M, Bozkurt B, et al. 2013 ACCF/AHA guideline for the management of heart failure: a report of the American College of Cardiology Foundation/American Heart Association Task Force on practice guidelines. Circulation 2013;128(16):e240-327.
3. Jencks SF, Williams MV, Coleman EA. Rehospitalizations among patients in the Medicare fee-for-service program. N Engl J Med 2009;360(14):1418.
4. Ross JS, Chen J, Lin Z, et al. Recent national trends in readmission rates after heart failure hospitalization. Circ Heart Fail 2010;3(1):97-103.
5. Heidenreich PA, Trogdon JG, Khavjou OA, et al. Forecasting the future of cardiovascular disease in the United States: a policy statement from the American Heart Association. Circulation 2011;123(8):933-44.
6. Go AS, Mozaffarian D, Roger VL, et al. Heart disease and stroke statistics-2013 update: a report from the American Heart Association. Circulation 2013;127(1): e6-245.
7. Roger VL, Weston SA, Redfield MM, et al. Trends in heart failure incidence and survival in a community-based population. JAMA 2004;292(3):344-50.
8. Kodiath M, Kelly A, Shively M. Improving quality of life in patients with heart failure: an innovative behavioral intervention. J Cardiovasc Nurs 2005;20(1):43-8.
9. Moser DK, Doering LV, Chung ML. Vulnerabilities of patients recovering from an exacerbation of chronic heart failure. Am Heart J 2005;150(5):984.
10. Schwarz KA, Elman CS. Identification of factors predictive of hospital readmissions for patients with heart failure. Heart Lung 2003;32(2):88-99.
11. Westlake C, Dracup K, Fonarow G, et al. Depression in patients with heart failure. J Card Fail 2005;11(1):30-5.
12. Bardia A, Arieas E, Zhang Z, et al. Comparison of breast cancer recurrence risk and cardiovascular disease incidence risk among postmenopausal women with breast cancer. Breast Cancer Res Treat 2012;131(3):907-14.

13. Hooning MJ, Botma A, Aleman BM, et al. Long-term risk of cardiovascular disease in 10-year survivors of breast cancer. J Natl Cancer Inst 2007;99(5):365–75.
14. Schonberg MA, Marcantonio ER, Ngo L, et al. Causes of death and relative survival of older women after a breast cancer diagnosis. J Clin Oncol 2011;29(12): 1570–7.
15. Mast ME, Heijenbrok MW, Petoukhova AL, et al. Preradiotherapy calcium scores of the coronary arteries in a cohort of women with early-stage breast cancer: a comparison with a cohort of healthy women. Int J Radiat Oncol Biol Phys 2011; 83(3):853–8.
16. Patnaik JL, Byers T, DiGuiseppi C, et al. The influence of comorbidities on overall survival among older women diagnosed with breast cancer. J Natl Cancer Inst 2011;103(14):1101–11.
17. Seidman A, Hudis C, Pierri MK, et al. Cardiac dysfunction in the trastuzumab clinical trials experience. J Clin Oncol 2002;20(5):1215–21.
18. Yeh ET, Bickford CL. Cardiovascular complications of cancer therapy: incidence, pathogenesis, diagnosis, and management. J Am Coll Cardiol 2009;53(24): 2231–47.
19. Curigliano G, Mayer EL, Burstein HJ, et al. Cardiac toxicity from systemic cancer therapy: a comprehensive review. Prog Cardiovasc Dis 2010;53(2):94–104.
20. Albini A, Pennesi G, Donatelli F, et al. Cardiotoxicity of anticancer drugs: the need for cardio-oncology and cardio-oncological prevention. J Natl Cancer Inst 2010; 102(1):14–25.
21. Volkova M, Russell R 3rd. Anthracycline cardiotoxicity: prevalence, pathogenesis and treatment. Curr Cardiol Rev 2011;7(4):214–20.
22. Sawyer DB, Zuppinger C, Miller TA, et al. Modulation of anthracycline-induced myofibrillar disarray in rat ventricular myocytes by neuregulin-1beta and anti-erbB2: potential mechanism for trastuzumab-induced cardiotoxicity. Circulation 2002;105(13):1551–4.
23. Campos EC, O'Connell JL, Malvestio LM, et al. Calpain-mediated dystrophin disruption may be a potential structural culprit behind chronic doxorubicin-induced cardiomyopathy. Eur J Pharmacol 2011;670(2–3):541–53.
24. Sawyer DB, Peng X, Chen B, et al. Mechanisms of anthracycline cardiac injury: can we identify strategies for cardioprotection? Prog Cardiovasc Dis 2010; 53(2):105–13.
25. Zuppinger C, Suter TM. Cancer therapy-associated cardiotoxicity and signaling in the myocardium. J Cardiovasc Pharmacol 2010;56(2):141–6.
26. Octavia Y, Tocchetti CG, Gabrielson KL, et al. Doxorubicin-induced cardiomyopathy: from molecular mechanisms to therapeutic strategies. J Mol Cell Cardiol 2012;52(6):1213–25.
27. Katz AM. Heart failure: a hemodynamic disorder complicated by maladaptive proliferative responses. J Cell Mol Med 2003;7(1):1–10.
28. Opie LH. Mechanisms of cardiac contraction and relaxation. In: Zipes DP, Braunwald E, Libby P, et al, editors. Braunwald's heart disease: a textbook of cardiovascular medicine. 7th edition. Philadelphia: WB Saunders Company; 2005. p. 457–89.
29. Struthers AD. Pathophysiology of heart failure following myocardial infarction. Heart 2005;91(Suppl 2):ii14–6 [discussion: ii31, ii43–8].
30. Ky B, Vejpongsa P, Yeh ET, et al. Emerging paradigms in cardiomyopathies associated with cancer therapies. Circ Res 2013;113(6):754–64.
31. Force T, Krause DS, Van Etten RA. Molecular mechanisms of cardiotoxicity of tyrosine kinase inhibition. Nat Rev Cancer 2007;7(5):332–44.

32. van Heeckeren WJ, Sanborn SL, Narayan A, et al. Complications from vascular disrupting agents and angiogenesis inhibitors: aberrant control of hemostasis and thrombosis. Curr Opin Hematol 2007;14(5):468–80.

33. Schimmel KJ, Richel DJ, van den Brink RB, et al. Cardiotoxicity of cytotoxic drugs. Cancer Treat Rev 2004;30(2):181–91.

34. Fainaru O, Adini I, Benny O, et al. Doxycycline induces membrane expression of VE-cadherin on endothelial cells and prevents vascular hyperpermeability. FASEB J 2008;22(10):3728–35.

35. Maitland ML, Bakris GL, Black HR, et al. Initial assessment, surveillance, and management of blood pressure in patients receiving vascular endothelial growth factor signaling pathway inhibitors. J Natl Cancer Inst 2010;102(9):596–604.

36. Zachary I. Signaling mechanisms mediating vascular protective actions of vascular endothelial growth factor. Am J Physiol Cell Physiol 2001;280(6): C1375–86.

37. Kamba T, McDonald DM. Mechanisms of adverse effects of anti-VEGF therapy for cancer. Br J Cancer 2007;96(12):1788–95.

38. Atzeni F, Turiel M, Caporali R, et al. The effect of pharmacological therapy on the cardiovascular system of patients with systemic rheumatic diseases. Autoimmun Rev 2010;9(12):835–9.

39. Voskuyl AE. The heart and cardiovascular manifestations in rheumatoid arthritis. Rheumatology (Oxford) 2006;45(Suppl 4):iv4–7.

40. Blum A, Miller H. Pathophysiological role of cytokines in congestive heart failure. Annu Rev Med 2001;52:15–27.

41. Rankin JA. Biological mediators of acute inflammation. AACN Clin Issues 2004; 15(1):3–17.

42. Torre-Amione G. Immune activation in chronic heart failure. Am J Cardiol 2005; 95(11A):3C–8C [discussion: 38C–40C].

43. Cacciapaglia F, Navarini L, Menna P, et al. Cardiovascular safety of anti-TNF-alpha therapies: facts and unsettled issues. Autoimmun Rev 2011;10(10): 631–5.

44. Sarzi-Puttini P, Atzeni F, Shoenfeld Y, et al. TNF-alpha, rheumatoid arthritis, and heart failure: a rheumatological dilemma. Autoimmun Rev 2005;4(3):153–61.

45. Chung ES, Packer M, Lo KH, et al. Randomized, double-blind, placebo-controlled, pilot trial of infliximab, a chimeric monoclonal antibody to tumor necrosis factor-alpha, in patients with moderate-to-severe heart failure: results of the anti-TNF Therapy against Congestive Heart Failure (ATTACH) trial. Circulation 2003;107(25):3133–40.

46. Mann DL, McMurray JJ, Packer M, et al. Targeted anticytokine therapy in patients with chronic heart failure: results of the Randomized Etanercept Worldwide Evaluation (RENEWAL). Circulation 2004;109(13):1594–602.

47. Popa C, Netea MG, Radstake T, et al. Influence of anti-tumour necrosis factor therapy on cardiovascular risk factors in patients with active rheumatoid arthritis. Ann Rheum Dis 2005;64(2):303–5.

48. Kaplan MJ. Cardiovascular complications of rheumatoid arthritis: assessment, prevention, and treatment. Rheum Dis Clin North Am 2010;36(2):405–26.

49. Danila MI, Patkar NM, Curtis JR, et al. Biologics and heart failure in rheumatoid arthritis: are we any wiser? Curr Opin Rheumatol 2008;20(3):327–33.

50. Piano MR. Alcoholic cardiomyopathy: incidence, clinical characteristics, and pathophysiology. Chest 2002;121(5):1638–50.

51. Piano MR, Phillips SA. Alcoholic cardiomyopathy: pathophysiologic insights. Cardiovasc Toxicol 2014;14(4):291–308.

52. Schwartz BG, Rezkalla S, Kloner RA. Cardiovascular effects of cocaine. Circulation 2010;122(24):2558–69.
53. Przywara DA, Dambach GE. Direct actions of cocaine on cardiac cellular electrical activity. Circ Res 1989;65(1):185–92.

Characteristics, Complications, and Treatment of Acute Pericarditis

 CrossMark

Janet A. Kloos, RN, PhD, MSN, CCNS, CCRN*

KEYWORDS

- Acute pericarditis • Retrosternal chest pain • Pericardial effusion

KEY POINTS

- Acute pericarditis is an inflammation of the pericardial sac occurring predominantly in men and in those aged 20 to 50 years.
- Approximately 65% to 85% of cases of pericarditis result from idiopathic viral or bacterial infections. Noninfectious causes are cardiac surgery, percutaneous coronary intervention, systemic inflammatory conditions, and renal failure.
- Classic history and physical findings are recent viral symptoms, chest pain, and pericardial rub.
- Diagnostic tests include echocardiogram, cardiac MRI or computed tomography scan, and laboratory blood tests such as antinuclear antibodies, erythrocyte sedimentation rate, and high-sensitivity C-reactive protein.
- Treatment includes use of colchicine, acetylsalicylic acid, and nonsteroidal antiinflammatory drugs.

INTRODUCTION

> **Case Study**
>
> Mr Edwards is a 40-year-old man admitted with sharp chest pain that worsens on inspiration and radiates to his left arm. He provides a history of fever, muscle aches, chest congestion, and cough for 2 weeks. His electrocardiogram shows ST segment elevation in all leads. His high-sensitivity C-reactive protein is 4 mg/dL and his white blood count is 12,000.

Acute pericarditis presents challenging features because there are similarities between other conditions and complications that must be recognized and treated, at times, with urgency. This article reviews the normal function of the pericardium, the

---

Disclosure statement: The author has nothing to disclose.
University Hospitals Case Medical Center, 11100 Euclid Avenue, Harrington Heart and Vascular Institute, Wearn 109-Mailstop 5057, Cleveland, OH 44106, USA
* University Hospitals Case Medical Center, 3512 Tuttle Avenue, Cleveland, OH 44111.
E-mail address: Janet.Kloos@UHhospitals.org

definition of acute pericarditis, characteristic symptoms, history and physical findings, diagnostic blood and imaging reports, and recommended treatment. Several Italian reports about research conducted with use of colchicine are reviewed; however, the dosages of medications provided are current dosages available in the United States.

STRUCTURE AND FUNCTION OF THE PERICARDIUM

The pericardium, a membranous sac surrounding the heart, consists of an outer fibrous layer and an inner serous layer separated by the pericardial cavity that contains approximately 45 mL of fluid.[1,2] Although normal cardiac function can be maintained in its absence, the pericardium serves several important functions.[2] The pericardium anchors the heart in the thorax, provides an immunologic barrier, and mediates effects of trauma to the heart.[3] Pericardial fluid provides lubrication for ease of movement as the heart contracts and twists within the mediastinum.[3,4] A plethora of nervous innervation exists in the pericardium, resulting in severe pain with inflammation.[3,4] Additionally, prostaglandins secreted by the pericardium serve to modulate cardiac reflexes and tone.[2–4]

DEFINITION OF ACUTE PERICARDITIS

Acute pericarditis is a common condition resulting from inflammation of the pericardium that occurs acutely or secondary to a systemic condition.[5] Acute pericarditis is generally self-limited in that symptoms resolve in response to treatment within days to weeks.[6,7] Pericarditis can result in an effusive or a constrictive condition:

- Effusive pericarditis is characterized by an increase in the amount of serous fluid accumulating in the pericardial space.[8] Cardiac tamponade, a dreaded and potentially life-threatening complication of pericarditis, may occur as accumulation of fluid compresses the cardiac chambers and prevents filling.[9]
- Constrictive pericarditis occurs when fibrosis and rigidity develops, usually a result of chronic pericardial inflammation that impedes left ventricular filling and reduces cardiac output.[8,9] Right-sided heart failure can be also be found with constrictive pericarditis.[1,9]

INCIDENCE

Although the incidence of acute pericarditis is unknown, up to 5% of visits to emergency departments for nonacute myocardial infarction chest pain may be related to pericarditis.[10] Recent reports state that approximately 90% of pericarditis in developed countries is postviral. Imazio and colleagues[11] reported the incidence of acute pericarditis as 27.7 cases per 100,000 of the population per year in an urban area of Italy. In developing countries such as sub-Saharan Africa there is a high prevalence of tuberculosis (TB); the incidence of pericarditis is 70% to 80%; and, in those with human immunodeficiency virus (HIV), it is equal to or greater than 90%.

CAUSES

Almost 90% of cases of pericarditis have a viral cause.[3,12] A wide variety of viruses have been implicated in the development of pericarditis with the most common being influenza, Coxsackie, Epstein-Barr, and human herpes virus-6.[4] Several investigators report an idiopathic cause because diagnostic testing can provide a low yield of confirmatory results.[2,4,8,9,11] More specific details of causative viruses include:

- Enterovirus, echovirus, adenovirus, cytomegalovirus, Epstein Barr virus, herpes simplex virus, influenza, parvovirus B19, hepatitis C, and HIV.[12]

- Enteroviral pericarditis occurs with seasonal epidemics of Coxsackie viruses A and B and echovirus infections.[12]
- Cytomegalovirus pericarditis is especially more predominant in patients who are immunocompromised either by a systemic condition or are taking antirejection medications after transplant.[12]
- Tuberculous pericarditis can be found in immunocompromised patients.[2,8]

The pathologic process occurring in acute pericarditis can be explained on a cellular level. Multiplication of the causative virus in the pericardium stimulates a cellular response and leads to inflammation.[8] In cases in which viral multiplication is absent, several viral genomic fragments can elicit an inflammatory response. Antibodies to the fragments have been discovered years after the initial case, which is thought to be reason for recurrence.[8,12]

Major medical conditions associated with acute pericarditis include systemic diseases such as autoreactive or immune-mediated diseases, neoplasms, uremia, previous myocardial infarction, aortic dissection, and chest wall trauma.[2,3] Dressler syndrome, a postmyocardial infarction–related pericarditis, has become rare in the era of the thrombolytic therapy.[13,14]

Surgical conditions such as previous cardiothoracic or thoracic surgery may contribute to development of acute pericarditis (**Table 1**).[2,3]

DIAGNOSIS

In obtaining the history, patients typically relate a prodrome of low-grade fever (less than 39°C), complaints of malaise, myalgia, and a nonproductive cough.[12] Sharp retrosternal chest pain that decreases when sitting forward and worsens with inspiration and when supine is a classic symptom.[1,3,8] Chest pain due to pericarditis may travel to bilateral trapezius muscle ridges or to the scapular ridges because the pericardium is innervated by both phrenic nerves to the anterior pericardium.[2,10,15] Patients who complain of neck or shoulder pain should point to the location to determine involvement of the trapezius.[10] The pain of acute pericarditis has also been described as

Table 1
Acute pericarditis causes

Causes of Pericarditis	Examples
Idiopathic	Cause not found
Viral, infections	Common: chest colds, pneumonia caused by echovirus or coxsackievirus, influenza Rare: TB or rheumatic fever
Predisposing conditions	Cancer (including leukemia) Immune disorders (lupus, rheumatoid arthritis, ankylosing spondylitis, systemic sclerosing periarteritis nodosa, Reiter syndrome) HIV and AIDS Hypothyroidism Kidney failure
Acute conditions	Myocardial infarction (acute or delayed) little Coronary artery bypass surgery Trauma to chest Radiation
Medication effects	Procainamide, hydralazine, phenytoin, isoniazid, and some drugs used to treat cancer or suppress the immune system

radiating to the neck, arms, or the left shoulder.[8] Conversely, some patients may experience little or no pain. This includes patients with rheumatoid arthritis, pericarditis due to TB, neoplasm, uremia, or postradiation.[3]

A classic finding with physical examination is a pericardial rub, heard as a squeaky sound with each contraction, which is best auscultated using the diaphragm of the stethoscope at the left sternal border during expiration with the patient sitting forward.[10,14,15] This classic rub is triphasic, attributed to atrial contraction, ventricular contraction, and ventricular relaxation.[8]

The pericardial rub is triphasic in 50%, biphasic in 33%, and monophasic in the remaining 13% of patients.[6]

Examination of patients with a severe pericarditis should include checking for pulsus paradoxus, a decrease in blood pressure by more than 10 mm Hg with inspiration, which may indicate the presence of cardiac tamponade.[1,10] Kussmaul's sign, an increase in jugular venous pressure with inspiration, is another sign of cardiac tamponade.[2] The Beck triad identifies the classic signs of tamponade consisting of jugular venous distention, hypotension, and muffled heart sounds.[1]

The predominant characteristic electrocardiogram (ECG) change occurring in acute pericarditis is elevation of the ST segment in all 12 precordial leads.[1] More specifically, ST-T wave changes are generally diffuse and evolve in time. The approximate timeframe in which ECG changes in acute pericarditis evolve is more than 2 weeks.[8] Approximately 50% of patients with acute pericarditis display these changes.[8]

Absence of Q waves, upwardly concave ST segments, and lack of T wave inversion that occurs in acute pericarditis distinguishes the ECG from changes occurring in myocardial infarction (**Fig. 1**).[2,13] According to Hoit,[1] 4 stages of ECG changes occur:

- Stage I: ST segment elevation with upward concavity occurs within several hours of onset of chest pain.
- Stage II: ST segment returns to baseline. T waves may appear normal or have low amplitude.
- Stage III: Inversion of T waves occurs, which may remain indefinitely, especially in patients with tuberculous, uremic, or neoplastic pericarditis.
- Stage IV: The ECG normalizes.

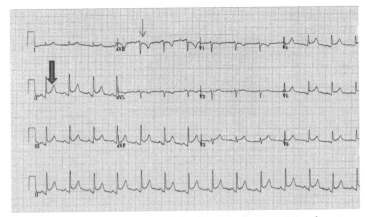

Fig. 1. "J" point depression in augmented lead aVR is characteristic of acute pericarditis (*arrow*). Diffuse concave ST segment elevation, seen in leads II, III (*large arrow*), augmented lead aVF, precordial leads V_3-V_6, are also characteristic. The P-R is subtly depressed in leads II, III, and V_3 to V_6.

Several imaging tests are useful in the diagnosis of acute pericarditis. The chest radiograph is usually normal in uncomplicated acute pericarditis.[2,8] In patients with moderate or large pericardial effusion, an enlarged cardiac silhouette may be found.[8] Evidence of TB, fungal disease, pneumonia, or neoplasm may also be found on chest radiologic examination.[12]

The use of 2-dimensional echocardiography is a class I recommendation for detection of acute pericarditis by the American College of Cardiologists, the American Heart Association, and the American Society of Echocardiography.[1,2] The 2-dimensional echocardiogram identifies pericardial effusion and confirms the diagnosis of acute pericarditis.[1,2,8] It also estimates the volume of fluid, identifies cardiac tamponade, may demonstrate cause of acute pericarditis, and can detect associated myocarditis.[1,2,8,9,16]

The computed tomography scan is a helpful diagnostic tool because it provides evidence of pericardial effusions, measures the size, geometry, and distribution of any effusion. It can also characterize the effusions as bloody, exudate, chyle, or serous.[1,2,12]

MRI can be used to estimate the volume of pericardial effusion, detects loculated pericardial effusion and pericardial thickening, and determines inflammation of the pericardium and presence of adhesions (**Fig. 2**).[1,2,11]

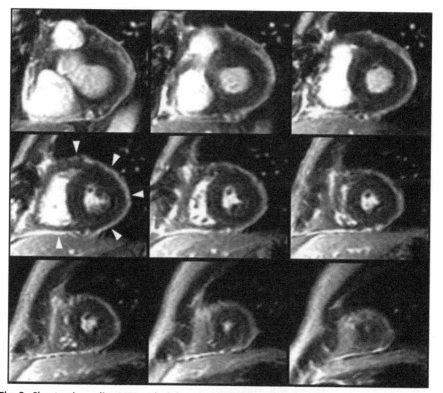

Fig. 2. Short-axis cardiac MRI with delayed gadolinium enhancement. In patients with acute pericarditis, notice the brightly enhanced pericardium (*arrowheads*) suggesting inflammation. (*From* Khandaker MH, Espinosa RE, Nishimura RA, et al. Pericardial disease: diagnosis and management. Mayo Clinic Proc 2010;85(6):576; with permission.)

Findings of serum laboratory tests are cited in the literature in the diagnosis of acute pericarditis. When evaluating the complete blood count, the presence of leukocytosis is determined.[17] Elevations in high-sensitivity C-reactive protein (hs-CRP) or erythrocyte sedimentation rate (ESR), and cardiac biomarkers can establish the diagnosis and guide prognosis and cause.[17]

Additional laboratory values that may be considered with suspicion for TB or malignancy can be evaluated with pericardial fluid aspiration.[8] Assessment of levels of pericardial fluid adenosine deaminase and carcinoembryonic antigen is important if there is suspicion for TB or malignancy-related pericarditis.[8] For patients with suspicion of a rheumatoid origin, a rheumatoid panel should be conducted, including antinuclear antibodies (ANA) and rheumatoid factor.[1,2,8] A screen for HIV should be performed with concern for immunologic deficiencies such as HIV and acquired immunodeficiency syndrome (AIDS) **(Table 2)**.[8,12]

Medications play a role in determining of the cause of pericarditis. Careful review of the patient's medication profile may alert the provider to potential causes of acute pericarditis due to unanticipated reactions. Patients on anticoagulation and thrombolytic therapy may convert an acute pericarditis to a hemorrhagic pericarditis.[12] Difficulty in distinguishing the reason for chest pain due to myocardial infarct or acute pericarditis may result in some patients being taken to the cardiac catheterization laboratory; given thrombolytics; and, therefore, converting to a hemorrhagic pericarditis.[3]

Maisch and colleagues[12] site additional medications that may induce pericarditis that follow the mechanisms occurring in the same manner as drug-induced lupus erythematosus. The culprit drugs are procainamide, tocainide, hydralazine, methyldopa, mesalazine, reserpine, isoniazid, and hydantoins. A drug-induced hypersensitivity

Table 2 Acute pericarditis findings	
Diagnostic Tests	**Suggestive Findings**
Chest radiography	Generally clear, cardiomegaly may be found with large pericardial effusion
MRI (CMR)	Most sensitive method for diagnosis Delayed enhancement of gadolinium uptake found in inflamed pericardium Estimates volume of pericardial effusion Detects myocardial involvement in myocarditis
2-Dimensional echocardiogram	Recommended in patients with acute pericarditis especially with hemodynamic compromise or concern for pericardial effusion.
ECG	Stage I: Diffuse ST segment with upward concavity initially Stage II: ST segments return to baseline with normal or low-amplitude T waves Stage III: Inversion of T waves, may occur indefinitely Stage IV: ECG normalizes
Cardiac computed tomography	Increased pericardial thickness may be seen but not diagnostic if not found Size, geometry, distribution of effusion seen
Blood tests	↑ESR, ↑ANA, ↑hs-CRP, ↑WBC, +blood culture, +HIV, +rheumatoid factors, +TB, ↑troponin I.

Upward arrows represent elevations in the related tests. The plus sign represents positive results.

Abbreviations: CMR, cardiac magnetic resonance; ESR, erythrocyte sedimentation rate; WBC, white blood count

reaction, idiosyncratic reaction, anthracycline derivatives, and other rare reactions can incite pericarditis.[12]

PROGNOSIS

The course of acute pericarditis is often benign because the occurrence of cardiac tamponade and constrictive pericarditis is rare.[9] Controversies about treating patients as outpatients versus hospitalization are reported in the literature.[11] Researchers studying acute pericarditis for several decades describe a profile of high-risk patients who should be treated in the hospital.[11] Independent predictors of high-risk patients include fever greater than 38°C, subacute course (symptoms occurring for several days or weeks), large pericardial effusion (diastolic echo-free space >20 mm width), or cardiac tamponade, immunosuppression; as well as failure to respond to aspirin or NSAID therapy.[11] Gender plays a role for those with greater risk for complications: women tend to have a higher prevalence of systemic and autoimmune diseases.[11]

Myocarditis may also be present in patients with acute pericarditis because they share similar causes.[9] Troponin elevation along with widespread ST segment elevation, representing subepicardial myocardial involvement, suggests myocarditis.[11] Differences in treatment exist between acute pericarditis and myocarditis. Guidelines for treatment of myocarditis should be used.[9,11]

Sequelae of acute pericarditis may provoke reevaluation of the prognosis. Incessant pericarditis is a relapse that occurs within 6 weeks of discontinuing or weaning of antiinflammatory medication. Recurrent pericarditis occurs after 6 weeks in 20% to 30% of patients who have been symptom-free.[11,17] Other sequela include refractory pericarditis, in which long-term high doses of corticosteroids (prednisone more than 25 mg per day) are required, and glucocorticoid dependence.[4]

CLINICAL MANAGEMENT

The treatment framework for acute pericarditis involves pharmacologic management, dietary and exercise restrictions, patient teaching, and follow-up with the health care provider.

Recognition of the underlying disease is key in determining the treatment regimen. For patients who have a postviral pericarditis, treatment is directed to resolve symptoms, prevent complications, and eradicate the causative virus. For example, in patients with cytomegalovirus virus, the pharmacologic approach is hyperimmunoglobulin once per day: 4 mL/kg on days 0, 4, and 8; and 2 mL/kg on days 12 and 16. For patients with HIV, TB, or fungal infections, current recommended regimens should be followed.[12] Maisch and colleagues[12] state that bacterial pericarditis is rare but fatal if untreated. Usually occurring as a secondary infection when infection occurs elsewhere in the body, bacterial endocarditis is included in the differential diagnosis when patients have preexisting pericardial effusions, immunosuppression, chronic diseases, cardiac surgery, and chest trauma.

Pharmacologic Management

Schwier and colleagues[4] emphasize the importance of appropriate drug therapy, achieving therapeutic levels, and a sufficient treatment course to obtain optimal clinical response. Inappropriate treatment can decrease quality of life and increase the risk for developing incessant, recurrent, or refractory pericarditis. The main drug classes for treatment of acute pericarditis are nonsteroidal antiinflammatory agents (NSAIDS), colchicine, and systemic corticosteroids.

Nonsteroidal antiinflammatory drugs

NSAIDS are first-line agents used to reduce inflammation and alleviate symptoms. The European guidelines recommend ibuprofen because side effects are rare and it promotes coronary artery blood flow.[10,12,16] The dosage of 300 to 800 mg every 6 to 8 hours, depending on the severity of symptoms, can be maintained for days or weeks until resolution of effusion. Schwier and colleagues[4] recommend avoiding indomethacin or ibuprofen in patients with heart failure and reduced ejection fraction (HFrEF). Gastrointestinal protection should be provided for all patients on NSAIDS.[4,8]

Aspirin (750 mg to 1000 mg) is suggested every 8 hours for 1 to 2 weeks for attack dose in the first occurrence of acute pericarditis and for 2 to 4 weeks if there is recurrence.[4] The aspirin dose should be tapered to twice daily every 1 to 2 weeks and then to once daily.[4] Aspirin is the NSAID of choice in patients with ischemic heart disease[4,11] patients developing pericarditis after acute myocardial infarction, aspirin is the preferred single agent.[8] Additional antiinflammatory drugs can impair scar formation in the setting of acute myocardial infarction and should be avoided.[3,4,12]

Another regimen recommended by the European guidelines is 50 mg of indomethacin 3 times daily for 1 or 2 weeks for first attack. With recurrence, continue for 2 to 4 weeks.[12] Schwier and colleagues[4] recommend 75 to 150 mg 3 times daily and then reduce the daily dose by 25 mg per day every 1 to 2 weeks.

Ketorolac tromethamine is recommended for pain management.[3,4,7] A black box warning advises that it should be used only as an extension of parenteral therapy and should be stopped at 5 days due to risk of gastrointestinal bleeding. The regimen starts with an oral dose of 10 mg per day every 4 to 6 hours, not to exceed 40 mg per day.[4] If parenteral routes are needed, the intramuscular dose is 30 to 60 mg once, or 15 to 30 mg every 6 hours.[4] Intravenous dosing is 15 to 30 mg every 6 hours (maximum daily dose is 120 mg).[4] Adjustments of dose is important for patients with renal dysfunction.[4]

Because NSAIDS can be irritating to the gastrointestinal system, especially when used for prolonged periods, gastrointestinal protection is warranted.[4,8,14] Patients with underlying gastrointestinal conditions or other conditions have an increased risk of toxicity or bleeding. These include history of peptic ulcer; age greater than 65 years; or concurrent use of acetylsalicylic acid, corticosteroids, or anticoagulants.[8] Proton pump inhibitors (omeprazole, pantoprazole) are the drugs of choice for gastrointestinal protection.[8,12]

Colchicine

Colchicine is a cornerstone class of pharmacologic agents in treatment of acute pericarditis. It interferes with mitosis in the cell nucleus and binds to tubulin, creating tubulin-colchicine complexes. Transcellular movement of collagen is inhibited, as well as various leukocyte functions, thereby providing antiinflammatory actions at low oral doses.[4,9,18,19]

The current recommended dosage is 1.2 to 1.8 mg as a single attack dose. The maintenance dose is 0.3 to 1.2 mg per day, which can be given as a single dose or 12 hours apart.[4] For initial pericarditis, colchicine should be continued for 3 months.[7] With recurrence, colchicine therapy should be maintained for 6 to 12 months.[4,7] Although symptoms of most patients resolve quickly with use of NSAIDS alone, current recommendations are to add colchicine to the NSAID regimen to reduce symptoms and to decrease the rate of recurrence.[16,17,20]

Use of colchicine is well tolerated, although some patients experience gastrointestinal symptoms such as nausea, vomiting, and diarrhea.[4,8] Other side effects, such as bone marrow suppression, hepatotoxicity, and myotoxicity, are less common.[11]

Chronic renal insufficiency can raise levels of colchicine, appropriate monitoring for side effects and lower dosage may be indicated.[8,11]

Colchicine is metabolized through the liver. Drugs that are metabolized through the cytochrome P450 isoenzyme system, such as cyclosporine, azole antifungals, ciprofloxacin, clarithromycin, propofol, isoniazid, protease inhibitors, may increase colchicine levels.[4,11] Colchicine was useful in reducing the incidence of primary pericarditis (OR 0.38, 95% CI 0.22–0.65) as well as recurrent pericarditis (OR 0.31, 95% CI 0.22–0.44). The most common side-effects were related to the gastrointestinal system and no severe adverse events were observed. Colchicine cessation either by the subject or physician was similar in both groups (OR 1.53, 95% CI 0.86–2.71).[21]

Avoiding grapefruit juice is recommended for patients taking colchicine although dosing adjustments are provided by the manufacturer for those who continue its use.[4] Schwier and colleagues[4] suggest reducing the dose of colchicine by 50% in patients over age 70.

Systemic corticosteroids

Steroids are indicated when patients have a connective tissue disease or autoreactive or uremic pericarditis. Prednisone is the drug of choice. The European guidelines suggest the early introduction of NSAIDs or colchicine in order to wean systemic steroids. Although the guidelines indicate use of intrapericardial steroids to avoid effects of systemic steroids, the level of evidence is B (small studies), class IIa (weight of evidence is in favor of usefulness or efficacy).[12]

Heparin

Although the European guidelines suggested cautious use of heparin, more recent studies did not find the use of heparin associated with increased risk of hemorrhagic pericardial effusion.[11]

Exercise Restrictions

Exercise restrictions include limitations of exercise and activity to that which is tolerable without worsening chest pain or shortness of breath.[11,12,22] A 2006 position paper suggests that after resolution of symptoms and normalization of biomarkers, such as hs-CRP, athletes should be temporarily excluded from competitive and amateur sports for at least 3 months.[22] If patients experience myocardial involvement, they should restrict participation according to the myocarditis recommendations.[22]

Follow-up Care

Patients with idiopathic or viral pericarditis without factors of high risk can be managed in an outpatient setting with follow-up visits at 7 to 10 days to evaluate response to treatment, at 1 month to check laboratory tests and hs-CRP, and afterward only if symptoms recur.[7,11] Patients being treated for acute pericarditis were found to have reductions in the inflammatory marker hs-CRP after 2 weeks, greater reduction at 3 weeks, and no presence at 4 weeks.[17] Patients exhibiting high risk for complications such as fever higher than 38°C, subacute onset, immunosuppression, trauma, oral anticoagulants, myopericarditis, severe effusion, or cardiac tamponade require hospitalization.[11]

Patient and Family Teaching

Patients and their families should be provided patient education materials from a reliable source such as UpToDate. This Web site has 2 types of patient education materials. "The Basics" is written in plain language at the fifth- to sixth-grade reading level and includes "Patient Information: Pericarditis in Adults (The Basics)" and "Patient Information: Pericarditis (Beyond the Basics)."

DISEASE COMPLICATIONS

Recurrence of pericarditis is the most common complication. On average, it occurs in 24% of patients.[2,23] Findings on physical examination, diffuse ECG ST elevations, and elevated markers of inflammation are similar to the first episode of acute pericarditis.[2,7] The characteristic midsternal chest pain that worsens when laying and lessens with leaning forward has been reported to be less than in the initial episode.[2] Treatment of recurrent pericarditis is similar to treatment of acute pericarditis and can be managed in the outpatient setting.[11] Two types of recurrence are cited are

- Intermittent: return of pericarditis chest pain after a symptom interval (usually more than 6 weeks)[2]
- Incessant: early reappearance of symptoms every time the patient is weaned from treatment.[2,23]

Constrictive pericarditis is a rare complication of chronic pericarditis. It is caused by thickening of the pericardium and characterized by adhesions or fibrosis causing compression of the atria and ventricles and inhibiting filling.[9,12] Reduced ventricular filling causes a resultant decrease in cardiac output and cardiac index. Right-sided heart failure may occur due to elevated filling pressures.[2] Signs of right-sided failure are characterized by marked jugular venous distension, hepatic congestion, ascites, and peripheral edema.[3] Exercise intolerance can progress to the development of muscle cachexia.[9]

Surgical removal of the entire pericardium has been the usual treatment of constrictive pericarditis.[7,12] Reports of 6% mortality in patients undergoing pericardectomy support careful consideration of this treatment.[7,12]

Pericardial effusion is another complication of pericarditis.[8,13] Small effusions generally resolve with standard treatment and patients are asymptomatic.[11,12] Moderate to large pericardial effusions are associated with specific diagnoses (in up to 90% of patients) such as neoplasms, TB, and myxedema.[11] Large pleural effusions not causing cardiac tamponade, without inflammatory signs, or a known medical cause generally result from a chronic idiopathic origin.[11]

Pericardiocentesis is not recommended unless pericardial effusions are large and develop quickly and/or cause cardiac tamponade as evidenced by diastolic right-sided collapse on echocardiography.[2,3,11]

Cardiac tamponade is a dreaded and potentially lethal complication of acute pericarditis if not recognized and treated.[2] In approximately 15% of patients with pericarditis, rapid accumulation of fluid can lead to cardiac tamponade.[2,3] Imazio and colleagues[24] found that 3% of subjects with recurrent pericarditis develop cardiac tamponade whereas 1 out of 296 subjects developed constrictive pericarditis. Physiologic deterioration occurs when extracardiac pressures reduce intracardiac volume filling, resulting in low cardiac output and hypotension.[3]

Treatment consists of pericardial drainage, the optimal treatment to remove fluid, can be performed in the setting of right heart catheterization to measure intracardiac pressures.[2,3] Echocardiographic-guided pericardiocentesis has been found to be safe.[11] A pericardial drain may be inserted to provide continued drainage to reduce the risk of recurrent effusion (**Fig. 3**).[2] Use of inotropic agents is controversial because endogenous adrenergic stimulation occurs.[2,3] Initiation of mechanical ventilation in a patient with cardiac tamponade contributes positive intrathoracic pressures, worsening impairment of cardiac filling, and sudden drop in blood pressure.[2]

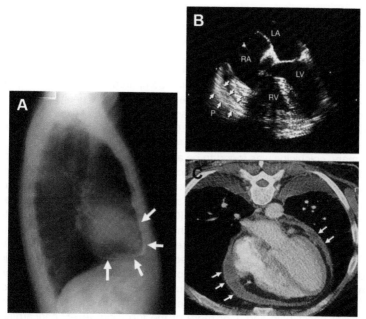

Fig. 3. Chest radiograph, transesophageal echocardiogram (TEE), and cardiac computed tomogram typical of constrictive pericarditis. (*A*) Pericardial calcification (*arrows*) on chest radiography is best seen from the lateral view over the RV and across the diaphragmatic surface of the heart. Pericardial calcification reflects chronicity of constrictive pericarditis and is associated with a higher surgical mortality. (*B*) Thickness of the pericardium is often difficult to determine by transthoracic echocardiography, but TEE is usually reliable in measuring the pericardial thickness (*arrows*). (*C*) Increased pericardial thickness (*arrows*) can be visualized on computed tomogram of the same patient. LA, left atrium; LV, left ventricle; RA, right atrium; RV, right ventricle. (*From* Khandaker MH, Espinosa RE, Nishimura RA, et al. Pericardial disease: diagnosis and management. Mayo Clin Proc 2010;85(6):588; with permission.)

CURRENT EVIDENCE

Guidelines for management of pericardial diseases had been supported by expert opinion and case studies. More recent studies have been conducted to provide research-based evidence.

Imazio and colleagues[20] conducted the Colchicine for Acute Pericarditis (COPE) trial to study the addition of colchicine to the conventional treatment of aspirin in subjects with acute pericarditis to verify safety and efficacy of colchicine as an adjunct and for prevention of recurrences. Inclusion criteria were (1) definite diagnosis of acute pericarditis (idiopathic, viral, and autoimmune causes), postpericardiotomy syndromes, and connective tissue diseases; (2) age equal to or greater than 18 years; and (3) ability to provide consent. Exclusion criteria were (1) tuberculous, neoplastic, or purulent causes; (2) known severe liver disease, blood dyscrasias, or gastrointestinal disease; (3) pregnant or lactating women and those not on contraceptive method; and (4) those with known hypersensitivity to colchicine or current treatment with colchicine.[20]

Subjects in group 1 were randomized to receive the standard aspirin dose of 800 mg orally every 6 or 8 hours for 7 to 10 days with gradual tapering over 3 to 4 weeks. Subjects in group 2 were treated with aspirin at the same dose while adding colchicine 1.0

to 2.0 mg for the first day and then a maintenance dose of 0.5 to 1.0 mg daily for 3 months. The sample was 120 subjects with 60 in each treatment arm.[20]

The results showed that subjects treated with aspirin alone were found to have a higher recurrence rate at 18 months compared with those with the addition of colchicine (32.3% and 10.7%, $P = .004$). Other findings were that symptoms were lower at 72 hours in the group with added colchicine compared with those on aspirin alone (11.7% vs 36.7%, $P = .003$). Logistic regression multivariate analysis found that use of corticosteroid was an independent risk factor for subsequent development of recurrences (OR 4.30, 95% CI 1.21–15.25, $P = .024$), whereas colchicine was found to be protective (OR 0.17, 95% CI 0.05–0.53, $P = .003$).[20]

In summary, colchicine was found to be a safe and effective addition to aspirin and provided evidence for reduction in recurrence of pericarditis. Side effects of colchicine were low, occurring in about 10% of cases, causing diarrhea, which resolved in lowering the dose and, in a small number of subjects, discontinuation was necessary.[20]

The Colchicine for Recurrent Pericarditis (CORP) trial was conducted to continue the research from the earlier trial. Because colchicine was found to be effective for secondary prevention of recurrent pericarditis, a second trial was conducted to evaluate the efficacy and safety as an adjunct in subjects with a first recurrence of pericarditis. The study was prospective, randomized, double-blind, and placebo-controlled.[17]

A sample of 120 subjects with a first recurrence of pericarditis was enrolled from 4 general hospitals in Italy. Recurrence of pericarditis was diagnosed in subjects who had recurrent chest pain and 1 or more of the following: fever, pericardial friction rub, electrocardiographic changes, echocardiographic evidence of new or worsening pericardial effusion or elevated leukocyte count, ESR, or hs-CRP level. Subjects were excluded if they had a first episode of pericarditis or second or subsequent episode of recurrence. Subjects were randomly assigned to receive placebo or colchicine in addition to aspirin, 800 to 1000 mg (or ibuprofen, 600 mg) orally every 8 hours for 7 to 10 days, with gradual tapering over 3 to 4 weeks.[17]

The procedure for colchicine dosing was the following: subjects received colchicine 1.0 to 2.0 mg on the first day, followed by maintenance dose of 0.5 to 1.0 mg per day for 6 months with 2 pills given 12 hours apart.[17]

Analysis of the data showed that the recurrence rate at 18 months in the colchicine group was 24% and 55% in the placebo group (absolute risk reduction 0.31 [95% CI 0.13–0.46], relative risk reduction 0.56 [CI 0.27–0.73], number needed to treat 3 [CI 2–7]). Colchicine significantly reduced the persistence of symptoms at 72 hours (absolute risk reduction 0.30 [CI 0.13–0.45], relative risk reduction 0.56 [CI 0.27–0.74]).

The highlight of the study was that addition of colchicine to aspirin therapy in recurrent pericarditis was halved at 18 months.

Ntsekhe and colleagues[23] studied the cytokine profile in 68 subjects with tuberculous pericardial effusion to determine the prevalence. Undiagnosed effusive constrictive pericarditis (ECP) carries high morbidity and mortality. It was postulated that subjects with effusive-constrictive pericarditis had a distinct cytokine profile that would aid in diagnosis.[23]

A sample of 91 subjects with suspicion for tuberculous pericarditis was evaluated. Subjects were excluded if hemodynamic data were unobtainable or were found to not have tuberculous pericarditis. The remaining 68 subjects with tuberculous pericarditis underwent intrapericardial and right heart catheterization, echocardiography, and laboratory analysis of cytokines in serum and pericardial fluid.[23]

Effusive-constrictive disease was found in half of cases of tuberculous pericardial effusion. It was characterized by greater elevation in the pre-pericardiocentesis right atrial pressure and pericardial and serum IL-10 levels. In multivariable regression analysis, right atrial pressure greater than 15 mm Hg (OR 48, 95% CI 8.7–265, $P<.0001$) and IL-10 greater than 200 pg/mL (OR 10, 95% CI 1–93, $P = .04$) were independently associated with effusive-constrictive disease.[23]

The researchers concluded that ECP occurs in half of cases of tuberculous pericardial effusion and is characterized by greater elevation in the pre-pericardiocentesis right atrial pressure and pericardial and serum IL-10 levels compared with subjects with effusive nonconstrictive tuberculous pericarditis.[23]

A prospective trial to identify risk factors for development of constrictive pericarditis (CP), an uncommon but potential complication of acute pericarditis, was conducted by Imazio and colleagues.[25] A sample of 500 men aged 51 plus or minus 16 years were studied.

Descriptive analysis showed that the causes of acute pericarditis were viral or idiopathic in 416 (83.2%) cases, followed by 36 (7.2%) cases of connective tissue disease or pericardial injury, 25 (5.0%) cases of neoplastic pericarditis, 20 (4.0%) cases of TB, and were purulent in 3 cases (0.6%). In a median follow-up time of 72 months (range 24–120 months), 9 of 500 (1.8%) subjects developed constrictive pericarditis. In subjects with idiopathic or viral pericarditis, 2 of 416 (0.48%) versus 7 of 84 (8.3%) subjects with nonviral or nonidiopathic causes developed constrictive pericarditis. Incidence of constrictive pericarditis according to pericarditis type was

- 52.74 cases per 1000 person-years were found for purulent pericarditis
- 31.65 cases per 1000 person-years for tuberculous pericarditis
- 6.33 cases per 100 person-years for neoplastic pericarditis
- 4.40 cases per 1000 person-years for connective tissue disease or pericardial injury syndrome
- 0.76 cases per 1000 person-years for idiopathic or viral pericarditis.

The researchers concluded that constrictive pericarditis is a rare complication of acute pericarditis except in bacterial or tuberculous cases.[25]

Zurick and colleagues[26] conducted a study of subjects with CP to determine evidence of pericardial delayed hyperenhancement (DHE) following administration of gadolinium contrast during cardiac magnetic resonance (CMR). The hypothesis was that pericardial DHE in subjects with CP would correlate with histopathologic findings of active inflammation. A sample of 25 CP subjects who underwent pericardiectomy following CMR-gadolinium study and 10 control subjects with no evidence of pericardial disease participated in the study.

Study results showed that 12 out of 25 (48%) of subjects with constrictive pericarditis were found to have DHE. CMR findings did correlate with inflammatory markers: greater fibroblastic proliferation and neovascularization, more chronic inflammation, and granulation tissue were found in subjects who were DHE positive. In addition, the DHE-positive group tended to have greater pericardial thickness.

The study concluded that the presence of DHE was associated with features of organizing pericarditis and may be a focus for future pharmacologic therapies.

The value of dynamic respiratory changes in left and right ventricular pressures in diagnosis of constrictive pericarditis was studied by Hurrell and colleagues.[27] Although echocardiography can demonstrate evidence of constrictive pericarditis, physiologic influences must be assessed to establish diagnosis. The purpose of the study was to evaluate the effectiveness of cardiac catheterization in diagnosing constrictive pericarditis by evaluating dynamic respiratory changes in left and right ventricular pressure relationships. Doppler echocardiography has shown increased transvalvular flow velocity in subjects with constrictive pericarditis.

The sample consisted of 36 subjects: 15 with postsurgical diagnosis of CP and 21 with heart failure.

Analysis of data found lack of sensitivity and specificity in measures obtained during cardiac catheterization failed to distinguish between CP and heart failure. Discordance between right ventricular and left ventricular pressures during inspiration, a sign of increased ventricular interdependence, accurately distinguished subjects in group 1 from those in group 2 ($P<.05$).

The researchers concluded that discordance between right and left ventricular pressures during inspiration, a sign of ventricular interdependence, accurately distinguished between subjects with constrictive pericarditis and those with heart failure. The study conclusion indicated that increased ventricular interdependence may be helpful in the diagnosis of CP in the cardiac catheterization laboratory.

SUMMARY

Acute pericarditis is an inflammatory condition that is most often related to a recent viral episode. A higher incidence of tuberculous pericarditis occurs in developing countries with a high prevalence of HIV or AIDS. Symptoms of a viral prodrome include low-grade fever, malaise, myalgia, and a nonproductive cough. A sharp retrosternal chest pain that worsens when supine and is alleviated when sitting forward is a characteristic symptom of acute pericarditis. Pericardial rub heard on auscultation is a classic physical finding. Examination of the patient for pulsus paradoxus or Kussmaul sign may alert the clinician of impending cardiac tamponade. Findings during history and examination, along with blood laboratory and diagnostic tests, are useful in determining the cause of acute pericarditis. Blood laboratory tests include hs-CRP or ESR, indicating inflammation; positive blood cultures or leukocytosis, indicating an infectious process; and other tests indicating the precipitating conditions of ANA and rheumatoid factor. Diffuse ST segment elevation and upward concavity are characteristic findings on 12-lead ECG. Additional diagnostic imaging useful in detecting acute pericarditis, the presence of pericardial effusion, or complications include chest radiography, 2-dimensional echocardiography, cardiac computed tomography, and CMR. Use of nonsteroidal antiinflammatory drugs, such as aspirin; ibuprofen; and, with caution, indomethacin and colchicine, are standard therapy. Treatment of autoimmune or immunodeficient conditions must be concomitantly provided. Use of colchicine has been found to reduce the recurrence. The course is generally limited to 2 to 4 weeks. Because the recurrence rate of acute pericarditis is high, vigilance in follow-up is key. There is a high recovery from uncomplicated acute pericarditis. Current evidence has identified prevalence, physical findings, and diagnostic tests to aid in the diagnosis of constrictive pericarditis.

REFERENCES

1. Hoit B. Diseases of the pericardium. In: Fuster V, Walsh R, Harrington R, editors. Hurst, the heart. 11th edition. New York: McGraw-Hill; Medical Pub Division; 2011. p. 1917–25.
2. Khandaker MH, Espinosa RE, Nishimura RA, et al. Pericardial disease: diagnosis and management. Mayo Clin Proc 2010;85(6):572–93.
3. Little W, Freeman GL. Contemporary reviews in cardiovascular medicine: pericardial disease. Circulation 2006;113:1622–32.
4. Schwier NC, Coons JC, Rao SK. Pharmacotherapy update of acute idiopathic pericarditis. Pharmacotherapy 2015;35(1):99–101.

5. Imazio M, Brucato A, Trinchero R, et al. Diagnosis and management of pericardial diseases: pericarditis. Nat Rev Cardiol 2009;6(12):743–51.
6. Tingle LE, Molina D, Calvert CW. Acute pericarditis. Am Fam Physician 2007; 76(10):1509–14.
7. Lilly LS. Treatment of acute and recurrent idiopathic pericarditis. Circulation 2013; 127:1723–6.
8. Sheth S, Wang D, Kasapis C. Current and emerging strategies for the treatment of acute pericarditis: a systematic review. J Inflamm Res 2010;3:135–42.
9. Farand P, Bonenfant F, Belley-Cote E, et al. Acute and recurring pericarditis: more colchicine, less steriods. World J Cardiol 2010;2(12):403–7.
10. Spodick D. Acute pericarditis: current concepts and practice. JAMA 2003;289: 1150–3.
11. Imazio M, Spodick D, Brucato A, et al. Controversial issues in the management of pericardial diseases. Circulation 2010;121:916–28.
12. Maisch B, Seferovic P, Ristic AD, et al. Guidelines on the diagnosis and management of pericaridal diseases. Eur Heart J 2004;25:1–28.
13. Chandavimol M, Cheung S, Ignaszewski A. Pearls and perils of acute pericarditis. B C Med J 2002;44(1):20–6.
14. Futterman LG, Lemberg L. Pericarditis. Am J Crit Care 2006;15:626–30.
15. Lang R, Hillis L. Clinical practice. Acute pericarditis. N Engl J Med 2004;351(21): 2195–202.
16. Imazio M, Trinchero R. Triage and management of acute pericarditis. Int J Cardiol 2007;118:286–94.
17. Imazio M, Brucato A, Cemin R, et al. Colchicine for recurrent pericarditis (CORP). Ann Intern Med 2011;155:409–14.
18. Adler Y, Findelstein Y, Guindo J, et al. Colchicine treatment for recurrent pericarditis. A decade of experience. Circulation 1998;97:2183–5.
19. Soler-Soler J, Sagrista-Sauleda J, Permanyer-Miralda G. Relapsing pericarditis. Heart 2004;90:1364–8.
20. Imazio M, Bobbio M, Cecchi E, et al. Colchicine in addition to conventional therapy for acute pericarditis. Results of the COlchicine for acute PEricarditis (COPE) trial. Circulation 2005;112:2012–6.
21. Raval J, Nagaraja V, Eslick G, et al. The role of colchicine in pericarditis–a systematic review and meta-analysis of randomised trials. Heart Lung Circ 2015;24(7):660–6.
22. Pelliccia A, Corrado D, Bjornstad H, et al. Recommendations for participation in competitive sport and leisure-time activity in individuals with cardiomyopathies, myocarditis and pericarditis. Eur J Cardiovasc Prev Rehabil 2006;12:876–85.
23. Ntsekhe M, Matthews K, Syed F, et al. Prevalence, hemodynamics, and cytokine profile of effusive-constrictive pericarditis in patients with tuberculous pericardial effusion. PLoS One 2013;8(10):e77532.
24. Imazio M, Trinchero R, Shabetal R. Pathogenesis, management, and prevention of recurrent pericarditis. J Cardiovasc Med 2007;8:404–10.
25. Imazio M, Brucato A, Maestroni S, et al. Risk of constrictive pericarditis after acute pericarditis. Circulation 2011;124(11):1270–5.
26. Zurick A, Bolen M, Kwon D, et al. Pericardial delayed hyperenhancement with CMR imaging in patients with constrictive pericarditis undergoing surgical pericardiectomy: a case series with histopathological correlation. JACC Cardiovasc Imaging 2011;4(11):1180–91.
27. Hurrell D, Nishimura R, Higano S, et al. Value of dynamic respiratory changes in left and right ventricular pressures for the diagnosis of constrictive pericarditis. Circulation 1996;93(11):2007.

High-Output Heart Failure Caused by Thyrotoxicosis and Beriberi

Brenda McCulloch, RN, MSN

KEYWORDS

- High-output heart failure • Thyrotoxicosis • Thionamides • Beriberi • Wet beriberi
- Shoshin beriberi • Thiamine deficiency

KEY POINTS

- High-output heart failure is less common than low-output heart failure and treatment options generally recommended for low-output heart failure may not be beneficial.
- Thyrotoxicosis causes many cardiovascular signs and symptoms, and can lead to high-output heart failure. Symptoms may not abate until the thyroid function has returned to near normal.
- Acute thiamine deficiency, or wet beriberi, can lead to high-output heart failure. Signs and symptoms include shortness of breath and marked peripheral edema. Patients at most risk for this include those with chronic alcoholism and malnutrition. Once thiamine administration is started, symptoms can rapidly improve.

INTRODUCTION

Heart failure is a complex clinical syndrome resulting from structural or functional impairment of ventricular filling or ejection of blood. This leads to symptoms of fatigue, dyspnea, and the retention of fluid. Disease of the pericardium, myocardium, endocardium, or heart valves can cause heart failure. Heart failure can also be caused by metabolic and nutritional abnormalities, such as severe hyperthyroidism and vitamin deficiency.[1] Heart failure is most commonly associated with a low-output state (cardiac index <2.5 L/min/m²),[2] but high-output heart failure may be seen in some patients. A high-output state has been defined as greater than 8 L/min or cardiac index greater than 3.9 L/min/m². In high-output heart failure, systemic vascular resistance is reduced because of vasodilation or systemic arteriovenous shunting.[3]

Current guideline recommendations for low-output heart failure treatment, such as vasodilators or positive inotropic agents, may not be appropriate for patients with

The author has no financial or commercial conflicts of interests and has received no funding for this project.
Sutter Medical Center, 2801 L Street, Sacramento, CA 95816, USA
E-mail address: mccullb@sutterhealth.org

high-output heart failure because they have low systemic vascular resistance and normal or near-normal ventricular contractility. Several disease states can cause high-output states, including sepsis, anemia, systemic arteriovenous fistulas, Paget disease, and multiple myeloma. Two additional causes of high-output heart failure include thyrotoxicosis and beriberi.[2] With prompt and complete treatment, both of these can be reversible. Thyrotoxicosis and beriberi leading to high-output heart failure are further described in this article.

THYROTOXICOSIS

Thyrotoxicosis is a syndrome caused by the inappropriate overproduction of thyroid hormone, leading to a hypermetabolic, hyperdynamic state. The excess production of thyroid hormones has a detrimental effect on the cardiovascular system. Such symptoms as resting tachycardia, breathlessness, and palpitations are some of the most prevalent. It is an acute disorder requiring prompt recognition and treatment. The association between thyrotoxicosis and heart failure has been well-established and long described in the literature.[4]

The most common cause of thyrotoxicosis is Graves disease, an autoimmune disorder responsible for up to 90% of cases of thyrotoxicosis.[5] Graves disease is more common in women than in men.[6] Thyrotoxicosis can also be caused by toxic multinodular goiter, toxic adenoma, thryoiditis, and excessive thyroid hormone replacement.[5,7] Thyrotoxic heart failure is more common in patients older than age 60.[8,9] It is more likely to occur when there is underlying cardiac disease; however, it can also occur when there is no cardiac disease. It has also been reported during pregnancy.[10]

Thyrotoxicosis can lead to thyrotoxicosis crisis, referred to as thyroid storm. It is not common and the important associated symptom includes hyperpyrexia. Body temperature can become elevated to 40.5°C to 41.1°C (105°F–106°F). Rapid treatment of thyroid storm in the hospital setting is essential.[6,11] Thyroid storm is beyond the scope of this article.

The Thyroid

The thyroid gland is located in the anterior neck behind the thyroid cartilage and its two lobes lie on either side of the trachea. The thyroid secretes two major hormones: tetraiodothyronince (thyroxin, or T_4) and triiodothyronine (T_3). Production of thyroid hormones is controlled by the hypothalamic-pituitary-thyroid axis, a complex feedback system (**Box 1**). T_4 is the predominant thyroid hormone accounting for about 80%

Box 1
Hypothalamic-pituitary-thyroid axis

Hypothalamus secretes thyrotropin-releasing hormone (TRH)

↓

TRH stimulates the anterior pituitary to secrete thyroid-stimulating hormone (TSH)

↓

TSH increases T_3 and T_4

Data from Elston MS, Conaglen JV. Thyrotoxicosis: pathophysiology, assessment, and management. J Prim Health Care 2005;32(6):407–13; and Dahlen R. Managing patients with acute thyrotoxicosis. Crit Care Nurse 2002:22(1);62–9.

of what is secreted, and T_3 accounts for the remaining amount. T_3 is the physiologically active form of thyroid hormone. T_4 is converted to T_3 in the liver, kidneys, and skeletal muscle. Circulating thyroid hormone is bound to plasma proteins.

Thyroid hormones increase the body's basal metabolic rate and have a direct effect on the heart and vasculature, and many other organs. Thyroid hormone has positive chronotropic and inotropic effects on the heart, increasing the heart rate and the heart contractility. Marked hemodynamic changes can occur and are listed in **Box 2**. Pulmonary hypertension is being recognized and reported in cases of thyrotoxicosis.[8,12] The reduced systemic vascular resistance present in high-output heart failure stimulates and activates the angiotensin-aldosterone axis, leading to increased absorption of sodium and water. This increases the circulating blood volume. Previously unknown valvular heart disease may be unmasked, leading to symptomatic mitral or tricuspid regurgitation.[11,12]

Signs and Symptoms of Thyrotoxicosis

The significant hemodynamic changes associated with thyrotoxicosis cause many of the symptoms the patient experiences. Common complaints of patients include feelings of breathlessness, tachycardia, palpitations, dyspnea on exertion, and/or orthopnea. They may also experience fatigue, diaphoresis or hot flashes, anxiety, nervousness, restlessness, tremor, heat intolerance, and frequent stools or diarrhea. They may note limited exercise tolerance, emotional lability, insomnia, or have recent unexplained weight loss.[8] If the patient has underlying coronary artery disease, they may have anginal chest pain.[13]

On physical examination, exophtalamos, or prominent bulging eyes, may be noted which is caused by swelling of the extraorbital muscles. The thyroid may be firm and nodules may be palpated. An audible bruit or a thrill may be palpable.[6] The skin is moist and warm and peripheral edema is common. A hyperdynamic precordium

---

Box 2
Hemodynamic findings in thyrotoxicosis

- Decreased diastolic arterial pressure
- Decreased systemic vascular resistance
- Decreased afterload
- Increased heart rate
- Increased stroke volume
- Increased cardiac output/cardiac index
- Increased systolic arterial pressure
- Increased contractility
- Increased diastolic relaxation
- Increased preload
- Increased left ventricular end-diastolic volume
- Increased left ventricular stroke work index
- Increased oxygen consumption
- Widened pulse pressure

Data from Refs.[5,8,12–14]

may be palpated and a systolic flow murmur, a snapping S1, loud S2, and an S3 heart sound may be ausculated. There are brisk carotid and peripheral arterial pulsations. Hyperreflexia may be present. Atrial fibrillation with rapid ventricular response may be found in up to 20% of patients with thyrotoxicosis and it is more likely to be present in men and the elderly. In the elderly patient population, apathetic thyrotoxicosis may be seen. This is a clinical syndrome associated with significant muscle weakness, weight loss, depression, and anorexia and many of the other typical symptoms of thyrotoxicosis may not be present.[2,6]

Diagnosing Thyrotoxicosis-Induced Heart Failure

Diagnosis of thyrotoxicosis is based on clinical findings and measurements of thyroid function tests. Key diagnostic findings include low levels of thyroid-stimulating hormone (TSH) and increased free T_3 and/or free T_4. See **Table 1** for additional details. The N-terminal pro–B-type natriuretic peptide is elevated because of the increased circulating blood volume leading to increased atrial size. Liver function tests, bilirubin levels, and alkaline phosphatase may also be elevated in the patient with heart failure.

Chest radiograph findings are consistent with heart failure and cardiomegaly may be noted. The electrocardiogram shows sinus tachycardia and a short PR interval may be present. A right bundle branch block may be present.[13] It is not uncommon to see atrial fibrillation with rapid ventricular response. Echocardiography may show preserved left ventricular function with an ejection fraction greater than 45%.[3]

Managing Thyrotoxicosis-Induced Heart Failure

The primary goal of treating heart failure caused by thyrotoxicosis includes adequately managing the symptoms of heart failure while quickly restoring normal thyroid function. β-Adrenergic blockers are initiated if there are no contraindications to their use to treat the symptoms of tachycardia, palpitations, tremor, anxiety, and heat

Table 1
Diagnosis of thyrotoxicosis

Test	Value	Finding	Rationale
TSH, serum	0.3–4.2 mIU/L	Deceased, may be immeasurable	Initial test of choice when hyperthyroidism is suspected. If the TSH is normal, the patient does not have hyperthyroidism. Elevation of thyroid hormones decreases TSH secretion by negative feedback from hypothalaumus
T4 by radioimmunoassay	4.6–12.0 µg/dL	Elevated	Overproduction of thyroid hormones
T3 by radioimmunoassay	80–230 ng/dL	Elevated	Overproduction of thyroid hormones
Free T4, serum	0.9–1.7 ng/dL	Elevated	—
Thyroid-stimulating immunoglobulin levels	≤1.3	Elevated in Graves disease	Elevated in autoimmune thyroid disease

Data from Rochester Test Catalog. Mayo Medical Laboratories: 2015. Available at http://www.mayomedicallaboratories.com. Accessed May 10, 2015; and Norman J. Thyroid gland function tests. EndocrineWeb. Available at: http://www.endocrineweb.com/conditions/thyroid/thyroid-function-tests. Accessed May 5, 2015.

intolerance. Propranolol (Inderal), a noncardioselective β-blocker, is commonly used. At high doses, propranolol blocks the peripheral conversion of T_4 to T_3. Patients with a history of asthma or chronic obstructive disease may benefit from the use of cardioselective β-blockers, such as atenolol or metoprolol (Lopressor, Toprol XL), that do not worsen restrictive airway disease. In the critical care setting, a continuous infusion of esmolol (Brevibloc), also a cardioselective β-blocking agent, may be used to control the tachycardia. Patients who cannot tolerate β-blockers may be treated with nondihydropyridine calcium channel blockers, such as verapamil (Calan) or diltiazem (Cardizem), to decrease heart rate. See **Table 2** for additional information about the use of β-blockers and calcium channel blockers.

Digoxin may be useful for some patients. Regular digoxin levels should be assessed. Loop diuretics, such as furosemide (Lasix), are given to promote diuresis and decrease fluid overload. Appropriate monitoring and replacement of potassium and magnesium is indicated.

Anticoagulation for patients with atrial fibrillation is important because the risk of thromboembolic events is increased. Vitamin K metabolism is increased in thyrotoxicosis and patients are more sensitive to warfarin (Coumadin). If warfarin is chosen for anticoagulation, careful monitoring of the protime/international normalized ratio (INR) is needed. The INR should be followed closely and the patient's treatment plan must be customized. If the patient is in atrial fibrillation, cardioversion should be deferred until thyroid function is normalized because the arrhythmia is more likely to recur while elevated thyroid hormone levels remain present.[5]

Primary therapies for returning the patient with Graves disease to a euthyroid or normal thyroid state include iodide and radioactive iodine therapy, antithyroid medication, and/or partial or total thyroidectomy. Removal of the thyroid may be delayed until medications have improved and stabilized the patient's symptoms.

Although it is more common today to use radioactive iodine and thionamide drugs, such preparations as potassium iodide (supersaturated potassium iodide) and Lugol solution may be administered. These solutions block the release of T_4 and T_3 within hours.

Radioactive iodine (^{131}I) is a safe and effective therapy, in common use since the 1940s for treating excess thyroid hormone production caused by Graves disease.[12] It is given as a capsule or an oral solution of sodium ^{131}I. It is rapidly absorbed and concentrated in the thyroid gland, destroying or ablating thyroid tissue within 6 to 18 weeks. Some patients, especially those with large goiters, may need a subsequent

Table 2
Use of β-blockers and calcium channel blockers

Medications	Nursing Implications
Propanolol, 10–40 mg PO every 6 h Atenolol, 25–100 mg PO daily Metoprolol, 25–50 mg PO every 6 h Esmolol, 50–100 μg/kg/min continuous infusion	In elderly patients, conservative initial doses are indicated, followed by careful dosage titration. In general, the elderly have unpredictable responses to β-blockers. Esmolol is recommended for use only in the critical care environment for severe thyrotoxicosis.
Verapamil, 40–80 mg PO every 8 h	Can be used for patients who do not tolerate β-blockers.
Diltiazem, 60–90 mg PO every 8 h	Can be used for patients who do not tolerate β-blockers.

Data from Refs.[5,7,12,15]

dose to adequately lower thyroid hormone levels. Radioactive iodine should not be used in pregnancy or lactation because it ablates the baby's thyroid gland. A pregnancy test should be obtained 48 hours before its use in any female with childbearing potential.[7]

Antithyroid medications, known as the thionamides, include methimazole (Tapazole) or propylthiouracil. Outside of the United States, carbimazole is commonly used. Thionamides act by blocking the synthesis of new thyroid hormones. Both of these medications have a narrow therapeutic window and require careful dosing. Methimazole is more commonly used but has the potential for teratogenic effects, so propylthiouracil is preferred for use in pregnancy. This therapy is usually maintained for up to 8 weeks and followed by radioiodine ablation or thyroidectomy or by continuing the drug therapy for a longer period of time. Before starting thionamides, and at each subsequent visit, the patient should be alerted to stop the medication immediately and call their physician when there are symptoms suggestive of agranulocytosis or hepatic injury.[7] See **Table 3** for additional information.

Thyroidectomy may also be recommended for patients with a large goiter. It is also recommended for patients who decline radioiodine or are allergic to thionamides. Whenever possible, patients with Graves disease undergoing thyroidectomy should be rendered euthyroid with methimazole before surgery. Potassium iodide should be given in the immediate preoperative period.[7] Thyroid storm may be precipitated by the stress of surgery, anesthesia, or thyroid manipulation and may be prevented by pretreatment with thionamides.

Amiodarone-Induced Thyrotoxicosis

A unique form of thyrotoxicosis can be induced by amiodarone (Cordarone, Pacerone), an iodine-rich class III antiarrhythmic drug commonly used to treat atrial and ventricular arrhythmias. One 200-mg dose of amiodarone corresponds to an intake of 75 mg organic iodide and generates 7 mg of free iodine. The normal dietary intake of iodine is only 100 to 200 μg daily, so daily dosing of amiodarone provides a large load of iodide to patients taking it.[18] Amiodarone can cause altered thyroid function and this effect can range from hypothyroidism to amiodarone-induce thyrotoxicosis. Patients on chronic amiodarone therapy should have TSH levels tested intermittently.

Amiodarone-induce thyrotoxicosis should be suspected when patients on amiodarone develop recurrent arrhythmias after a period of stability, or have unexplained weight loss or fatigue.[12,18] Amiodarone-induced thyrotoxicosis is confirmed when the TSH is low with normal or elevated free T_4 and free T_3 levels, negative thyroid-stimulating immunoglobins, and low or absent tracer uptake on thyroid scan.[5] Amiodarone should be discontinued when possible. Treatment with corticosteroids in combinations with thionamides may be beneficial in treating amiodarone-induced thyrotoxicosis. Radioactive iodine treatment may not be effective because the high iodide plasma concentration suppresses iodine uptake in the thyroid. Subtotal thyroidectomy may be needed for patients with large goiters, malignant nodules, or severe hyperthyroidism that does not respond to conservative therapy.[5,18]

BERIBERI

Beriberi is caused by severe thiamine (vitamin B_1, also spelled thiamin) deficiency lasting more than 3 months. Although not common in the United States, it is most commonly seen in patients with chronic alcoholism or those with poor nutritional status when there is inadequate thiamine replacement, including patients with eating disorders[19] or extreme dieting, prolonged enteral nutrition, or following bariatric weight

Table 3
Antithyroid medications

Medications	
Methimazole (Tapazole), 60–80 mg daily. First-line thionamide for most patients. Potentially teratogenic; do not use in pregnancy. Propylthiouracil, 500–1000 mg load, then 250 mg every 4 h. Preferred over methimazole in pregnancy, life-threatening thyrotoxicosis (thyroid storm), and adverse reactions to methimazole.	Side effects are dose related. Generally well tolerated but can cause side effects including nausea, vomiting, pruritus, rash, urticaria, arthralgias, arthritis, fever, and abnormal taste sensation. Agranulocytosis is a rare but serious complication of therapy that usually occurs within the first 60 d of therapy. Aplastic anemia and hepatotoxicity are other rare complications of thionamide therapy.
Sodium iodine 131 (^{131}I). One-time dose successful in most patients.	Destroys, or ablates, thyroid cells. Risk of hypothyroidism. Gastric distress can be a common side effect. Can cause a hypersensitivity reaction: angioedema; cutaneous and mucosal hemorrhage; and signs and symptoms similar to serum sickness, such as fever, arthralgia, lymphadenopathy, and eosinophilia. Women of childbearing ages should have a pregnancy test before receiving this drug. Do not use if patient is pregnant or lactating, or if planning pregnancy in the next 6 mo because it ablates fetal thyroid tissue.
Potassium iodide (supersaturated potassium iodide), 50 mg iodide/per drop PO 1–2 drops every 8 h. Potassium iodide-iodine solution (Lugol solution) 5–7 drops PO every 8 h. Lugol solution can also be added to an intravenous solution or can be given rectally.	Do not give until at least 1 h after antithyroid drugs, monitor for allergic reaction, dilute with juice or water. Side effects include nausea, vomiting, diarrhea, metallic taste. Allergic reaction uncommon.
Corticosteroids Hydrocortisone, 100 mg intravenous every 8 h. Dexamethasone, 2 mg intravenous every 6 h.	Inhibits the conversion of T_4 to T_3.
Cholestyramine, 4 g four times daily.	May be added when methimazole is used because it lowers serum T_4 and T_3 more rapidly than methimazole alone.
Lithium carbonate, 300 mg PO every 8 h.	Inhibits the release of thyroid hormones. Can be used if the patient cannot take thionamides.

Data from Refs.[7,16,17]

loss surgery.[20] There is also another form of alcohol-induced cardiomyopathy that is seen and is not related to thiamine deficiency, nor is it affected by the administration of thiamine.[1,21] Beriberi is more common in Asia, where a major component of diet is polished white dehusked rice, which is lacking in thiamine. It has also been reported internationally in prisoner of war camps, refugee camps, detention centers, and prisons where poor nutrition is present. There are two types of beriberi that may be seen in patients with acute thiamine deficiency: dry and wet.

Dry Beriberi

In dry beriberi, neurologic abnormalities predominate and the patient has peripheral neuropathy, sensory and motor deficiencies of the extremities, and muscle pain with atrophy. Severe dry beriberi can lead to the Wernicke-Korsakoff syndrome, a serious encephalopathy characterized by delirium, oculomotor abnormalities, and ataxia.

Wet Beriberi

Wet beriberi is associated with predominant cardiovascular symptoms and heart failure. There may also be neurologic symptoms in wet beriberi, but cardiovascular effects are more pronounced. Patients have marked peripheral edema, fatigue, dyspnea, and palpitations. A gallop rhythm may be noted. Systolic and diastolic murmurs may be present. Right heart failure predominates and jugular venous distention and ascites may be present. Hemodynamic changes seen in wet beriberi are listed in **Box 3**.[21] The most severe form of wet beriberi is referred to as Shoshin beriberi. These patients have hypotension, severe right and left heart failure, metabolic acidosis, and cyanosis leading to cardiovascular collapse. Shoshin beriberi can be fatal if not promptly recognized and aggressively treated.[22]

About Thiamine

Thiamine is an essential water-soluble vitamin, first discovered in 1926. It was named vitamin B_1 because it was the first of the B vitamins to be identified. Thiamine is a cofactor required for the synthesis of energy and is involved in a variety of glucose metabolism–related and neurologic functions.[19] It is important in carbohydrate metabolism, synthesis of nucleic acids and nucleotides, transport of ions of sensory and motor activity and nervous functions, synthesis of neurotransmitters, and cognitive function.[20]

Thiamine is commonly found in enriched, fortified, and whole grain products, such as bread and cereals, and pasta; beef, lean pork, organ meats, and eggs; legumes, peas, nuts, and seeds. Thiamine storage in the body is limited to about 30 mg, which can be completely depleted within 20 days of inadequate intake, making regular intake

---

Box 3
Hemodynamic findings in wet beriberi

- Decreased systemic vascular resistance
- Decreased afterload
- Increased cardiac output (as high as 20 L/min reported)
- Increased cardiac index
- Increased stroke volume
- Increased venous return
- Increased right heart pressures
- Wide pulse pressure

Data from Gubbay ER. Beriberi heart disease. Can Med Assoc J 1966;95:21–7.

of thiamine-rich foods important to ensure healthy nutrition.[20] The body is readily depleted of thiamine by fever and other metabolic stress.

The recommended daily allowance for thiamine is 1.2 mg daily for males, 1.1 mg daily for females, and 1.4 mg daily during pregnancy and lactation.[23] Thiamine is absorbed from food in the small intestine with maximum absorption occurring in the proximal jejunum.[20] A high alcohol intake contributes to thiamine deficiency by decreasing the transport of thiamine across the intestinal mucosa.

Signs and Symptoms of Wet Beriberi

In severe thiamine deficiency, peripheral vasodilation occurs, leading to a high state. Hemodynamic changes seen in wet beriberi are listed in **Box 3**. This leads to salt and water retention mediated through the renin-angiotensin-aldosterone system in the kidneys. As the vasodilation progresses, the kidneys detect a relative loss of volume and respond by conserving sodium leading to increased circulating volume.

In classic wet beriberi, patients complain of fatigue and malaise and signs and symptoms include shortness of breath, and/or paroxysmal nocturnal dyspnea. On physical examination, marked peripheral edema of the lower extremities is common. Elevated jugular venous pressure is present.

Diagnosing Wet Beriberi

The diagnosis of wet beriberi requires a high degree of suspicion and should be considered when evaluating patients with the abrupt onset of heart failure who have a history of alcoholism and/or poor nutrition.[24] Diagnostic criteria for wet beriberi published initially in 1945 include cardiomegaly with normal sinus rhythm, dependent edema, elevated jugular venous pressure, signs of neuritis and/or pellegra (hyperpigmented rash, red tongue caused by niacin deficiency), nonspecific ST-T wave changes on the electrocardiogram, no other cause of heart disease, gross deficiency of thiamine for 3 or more months, with improvement in heart size after thiamine therapy.[25]

Thiamine levels will be low. Additional laboratory testing may show low serum proteins, elevated blood urea nitrogen, and elevated pyruvate and lactate levels. Troponin I may also be elevated because of heart failure. Concomitant nutritional anemia is also common, so hemoglobin and hematocrit levels may be low. Serum lactate may be elevated. Magnesium levels may be low. The liver may also be affected if the cause of the beriberi is heavy alcohol intake, resulting in elevated protime/INR, and decreased albumin, calcium, and phosphate.

The chest radiograph demonstrates heart failure and enlargement of the right atria and ventricle. In some patients there may also be left ventricular enlargement. The electrocardiogram may show sinus tachycardia and nonspecific ST-T wave changes.

Treating Wet Beriberi

Thiamine replacement is essential in treating wet beriberi and initial dosing may range from 100 to 500 mg intravenously, followed by 25 to 100 mg orally daily for at least 2 weeks. Empiric treatment with thiamine may be given for patients with acute-onset heart failure who have a history of alcoholism or poor nutrition. Thiamine is a water-soluble vitamin and excess amounts are excreted by the kidney.[26] Rapid improvements in the patient's condition can be seen within hours of bolus dosing of thiamine.

Nutritional anemia is commonly also present in beriberi and treatment of it is needed. Oral multivitamin supplementation may be considered: thiamine, 100 mg; pyridoxine (vitamin B$_6$), 2 mg; folic acid, 400 μg to 1 mg[26]; and the administration of supplemental iron.

Careful use of diuretic therapy is indicated to treat the heart failure and decrease extra circulating volume. Typically, after adequate treatment with thiamine and diuretics, heart failure abates and heart size returns to normal.

CARING FOR THE PATIENT WITH HIGH-OUTPUT HEART FAILURE CAUSED BY THYROTOXICOSIS OR BERIBERI

Patients with high-output heart failure caused by either thyrotoxicosis or wet beriberi can be very ill and present to the hospital because of fluid overload and shortness of breath.

For the patient in heart failure, it is essential to provide adequate ventilation and oxygenation. Assess respiratory status regularly. Provide supplemental oxygenation as ordered, especially if the patient is experiencing dyspnea. The patient may be more comfortable with the head of the bed elevated. Continuous cardiac monitoring may be indicated because tachycardia and atrial arrhythmias may be present. Some patients may benefit from hemodynamic monitoring in the critical care unit while the diagnosis is confirmed and the treatment plan is developed.

Rapid management of fluid overload is needed; loop diuretics are indicated for many of these patients. Careful monitoring of fluid status and replacement of electrolytes is needed. Daily weights may be indicated while the patient is on diuretic therapy.

Provide regular oral care. Alcoholic patients may have glossitis, or inflammation of the tongue, and patients with beriberi may have pellagra, affecting their mouth. Regular oral care also decreases the risk of hospital-acquired pneumonia. Assessment of skin integrity is needed regularly and the patient should be repositioned often. Venous thromboembolism prophylaxis is initiated.

Provide reassurance; promote a calm and quiet environment. Anxiety abates as treatment of the high-output heart failure and thyrotoxicosis or beriberi is continued. Rest periods are important because fatigue and activity intolerance is common. They may also have been experiencing insomnia. Reduce stimuli and allow for uninterrupted rest periods. When talking with the patient, use active listening.

Administer medications as ordered for the underlying cause of the high-output heart failure and monitor for side effects. During the patient's hospitalization, teach them about their medications because some of them will be continued after discharge from the hospital.

Monitor for hypoglycemia because gluconeogensis can be activated. Monitor the fasting blood glucose. Perform point-of-care testing with a glucometer as ordered.

A thorough dietary assessment is needed for patients. A consultation with a dietitian is beneficial. Weight loss is common in thyrotoxicosis; and poor nutrition, anemia, and muscle wasting can be seen in beriberi, especially in those with chronic alcoholism who are often deficient in thiamine, folate, iron, and vitamin B$_6$.[27] Provide supplemental feedings high in protein and calories. Supplemental multivitamins are commonly prescribed.

Fever caused by the hypermetabolic state of thyrotoxicosis may be present and may need treatment with acetaminophen or active cooling with a cooling blanket. Aspirin should be avoided because it can increase the conversion of T$_4$ to T$_3$.

Patients with exopthalmos caused by Graves disease may have eye discomfort and sensitivity to light. A darkened environment is helpful, in addition to artificial tears, eye lubricant, eye patches, or sunglasses.

Teach the patient and their family about their underlying condition. For the alcoholic patient, discuss the benefits of a healthy diet, good sources of thiamine, and the benefits of decreased alcohol intake. A social work consultation may be helpful for the patient seeking assistance with their alcoholism.

SUMMARY

High-output heart failure has several causes, including thyrotoxicosis and beriberi. Although not commonly seen the United States, these disorders may be seen in the outpatient clinic, emergency department, or critical care units, depending on the extent of the patient's symptoms. The clinical manifestations of both have been described. Prompt recognition assists in guiding the medical management and nursing care to return the patient to pre-high-output heart failure state.

REFERENCES

1. Yancy CW, Jessup M, Bozkurt B, et al. 2013 ACCF/AHA guideline for the management of heart failure: a report of the American College of Cardiology Foundation/American Heart Association Task Force on practice guidelines. Circulation 2013;128:e240–327.
2. Givertz MM, Haghighat A. High-output heart failure. Waltham (MA): UpToDate; 2012. Available at: http://www.uptodate.com/contents/high-output-heart-failure?source=search_result&search=high+output+heart+failure&selectedTitle=1%7E53. Accessed May 6, 2015.
3. Mehta PA, Dubrey SW. High output heart failure. Q J Med 2009;102:235–41.
4. Kolawole BA, Balogun MO. Thyrotoxicosis and the heart: a review of the literature. Niger J Med 2001;10(2):50–4.
5. Roffi M, Cattaneo F, Topol EJ. Thyrotoxicosis and the cardiovascular system: subtle but serious effects. Cleve Clin J Med 2003;70(1):57–63.
6. Elston MS, Conaglen JV. Thyrotoxicosis: pathophysiology, assessment, and management. J Prim Health Care 2005;32(6):407–13.
7. Bahn RS, Burch HB, Cooper DS, et al. Hyperthyroidism and other causes of thyrotoxicosis: management guidelines of the American Thyroid Association and the American Association of Clinical Endocrinologists. Thyroid 2011;21(6): 593–646.
8. Klein I. Cardiovascular effects of hyperthyroidism. Waltham (MA): UpToDate; 2014. Available at: http://www.uptodate.com/contents/cardiovascular-effects-of-hyperthyroidism?source=search_result&search=cardiovascular+effects+of+hyperthyroidism&selectedTitle=1%7E150. Accessed May 6, 2015.
9. Woeber KA. Thyrotoxicosis and the heart. N Engl J Med 1992;327:94–8.
10. Sheffield JS, Cunningham EG. Thyrotoxicosis and heart failure that complicate surgery. Am J Obstet Gynecol 2004;190:211–7.
11. Dahlen R. Managing patients with acute thyrotoxicosis. Crit Care Nurse 2002; 22(1):62–9.
12. Dahl P, Danzi S, Klein I. Thyrotoxic cardiac disease. Curr Heart Fail Rep 2008;5: 170–6.
13. Fadel BM, Ellahham S, Ringel MD, et al. Hyperthyroid heart disease. Clin Cardiol 2000;23:402–8.
14. Vargas-Uriocoechea H, Bonelo-Perdomo A, Sierra-Torres CH. Effects of thyroid hormones on the heart. Clin Investig Arterioscler 2014;26(6):296–309.

15. Thyrotoxicosis. In: Clinical pharmacology. 2015. Available at: http://www. clinicalpharmacology-ip.com/Forms/AdvSearch/indsearch.aspx?sec=indi&i= 746879726f746f7869636f736973. Accessed May 5, 2015.

16. Drugs and Supplements: Methimazole. In Mayo Clinic for Health Professionals 2015. Available at: http://www.mayoclinic.org/drugs-supplements/methimazole-oral-route/before-using/drg-20073004. Accessed May 5, 2015.

17. Ross DS. Pharmacology and toxicity of thionamides. Waltham (MA): UpToDate; 2015. Available at: http://www.uptodate.com/contents/pharmacology-and-toxicity-of-thionamides?source=search_result&search=pharmacology+and+toxicity+ of+thionamides&selectedTitle=1%7E150. Accessed May 14, 2015.

18. Roffi M, Cattaneo F, Brandle M. Thyrotoxicosis and the cardiovascular system. Minerva Endocrinol 2005;90(2):47–58.

19. Ward KE, Happel KI. Case report: an eating disorder leading to wet beriberi heart failure in a 30 year old woman. Am J Emerg Med 2013;13:460.e5–6.

20. Stroh C, Meyer F, Manger T. Beriberi, a severe complication after metabolic surgery: review of the literature. Obes Facts 2014;7:246–52.

21. Gubbay ER. Beriberi heart disease. CMAJ 1966;95:21–7.

22. Dabar G, Harmouche C, Habr B, et al. Shoshin beriberi in critically-ill patients: case series. Nutr J 2015;14:51.

23. Pazirandeh S, Lo CW, Burns DL. Overview of water soluble vitamins. Waltham (MA): UpToDate; 2014. Available at: http://www.uptodate.com/contents/ overview-of-water-soluble-vitamins?source=search_result&search=overview+ of+water+soluble+vitamins&selectedTitle=1%7E150. Accessed May 6, 2015.

24. Chisolm-Straker M, Cherkas D. Altered and unstable: wet beriberi, a clinical review. J Emerg Med 2013;45(3):341–4.

25. Jones RH. Beriberi heart disease. Circulation 1959;19:275–83.

26. Beriberi. In: Clinical pharmacology. 2015. Available at: www.clinical pharmacology.com. Accessed May 5, 2015.

27. Gramlich L, Tandon P, Rahman A. Nutritional status in patients with sustained heavy alcohol use. Waltham (MA): UpToDate; 2014. Available at: http://www. uptodate.com/contents/nutritional-status-in-patients-with-sustained-heavy-alcohol-use?source=search_result&search=nutritional+status+in+patients+with+ sustained+alcohol&selectedTitle=1%7E150. Accessed May 11, 2015.

Sleep and Heart Failure

Kimberly A. Nelson, DNP, RN-BC, ACNS-BC, CHFN, CCPC, CCRP, RDCS[a],
Robin J. Trupp, PhD, RN, ACNP-BC, CHFN[b],*

KEYWORDS

- Obstructive sleep apnea • Central sleep apnea • Sleep-disordered breathing
- Heart failure • Noninvasive ventilator support

KEY POINTS

- Sleep-disordered breathing (SDB) is frequently undiagnosed and untreated in heart failure.
- Due to its high prevalence and poor outcomes, active recognition and treatment are warranted.
- Early recognition and prompt treatment of SDB has the potential to reduce health care expenses and mitigate the development and progression of cardiovascular disease.

INTRODUCTION

Sleep was once thought to be a passive part of daily life: a time in which the body and brain were inactive. It is now known the brain remains very active during sleep, and the importance of sleep on optimal health and physical and mental performance is more appreciated. In fact, sleep should be restorative, allowing the body and brain to recover from activities of the previous day and to prepare for the next. Yet, sleep deprivation is endemic in the United States and has recently been called a "public health epidemic" by the Centers for Disease Control and Prevention.[1] The exact amount of sleep needed varies by individual and age, but the National Institutes of Health recommends at least 10 hours of sleep daily for school-age children, 9 to 10 hours for teenagers, and 7 to 8 hours for adults.[2] However, the National Health Interview Survey reported in 2014 that nearly 30% of adults averaged less than 6 hours of sleep.[3] Additionally the National Sleep Foundation reported, despite rating sleep as "extremely important" for their own and their children's health, parents failed to set good examples for sleep, enforce bedtime rules, or limit electronics in the bedroom.[2]

Sleep deprivation can be either acute or chronic in nature, as in jet lag or routinely working night shift, caused by developmental stages, as in having young children, related to societal factors, like hectic schedules or constant electronic connectivity,

[a] Virginia Commonwealth University Medical Center, 1250 E Marshal Street, Richmond, VA 23219, USA; [b] University of Illinois at Chicago, College of Nursing, 845 S Damien Street, Chicago, IL 60612, USA
* Corresponding author.
E-mail address: rjtrupp@uic.edu

Crit Care Nurs Clin N Am 27 (2015) 511–522
http://dx.doi.org/10.1016/j.cnc.2015.07.008
0899-5885/15/$ – see front matter © 2015 Elsevier Inc. All rights reserved.

or result from poor sleep quality. Regardless, all produce reduced alertness, impaired concentration, and delayed reaction times. However, those with chronic sleep deprivation are more likely to develop hypertension, diabetes, depression, heart failure, or arrhythmias and experience increased mortality or decrements in quality of life and productivity.[4,5]

A frequent cause of poor sleep quality is sleep-disordered breathing (SDB), a disorder characterized by abnormalities in either the quality or quantity of respirations during sleep. In a population-based sample of adults aged 30 to 70, estimates are approximately 13% of men and 6% of women have moderate to severe SDB.[6] This represents a double-digit percentage increase from the previous decade, with obesity identified as a strong causal factor. In those with cardiovascular disease (CVD), the estimates of SDB are much higher, affecting 30% to 80% of hypertensive patients, 30% to 60% of patients with ischemic heart disease, and 50% to 80% of those with heart failure (HF).[5] Despite the high prevalence associated with SDB, attention, recognition, and treatment of this disorder are inadequate.

SLEEP PHYSIOLOGY

Sleep is a state of unconsciousness during which the brain is more responsive to internal, rather than external, stimuli.[7] Sleep is divided into non–rapid eye movement (NREM) and rapid eye movement (REM) stages. NREM makes up 80% to 85% of total sleep time and begins with stage 1 (the transition between wakefulness and sleep; also known as drowsiness), advances to stage 2 (decreased movement and fading of conscious awareness of the surroundings), and progresses to deeper sleep in stage 3.[8] During stage 3, the sleeper is totally unaware of the environment. Driven primarily by decreased metabolic needs, the respiratory rate declines, producing a rise in $Paco_2$, and parasympathetic nervous tone increases, such that heart rate and blood pressure are at their lowest. Brief arousals from sleep, lasting 3 to 15 seconds, result in a change to a lighter stage of NREM sleep but are not remembered by the sleeper. Because most time is spent in NREM, sleep should be a period of hemodynamic and cardiovascular tranquility.

The deepest level of relaxation follows NREM in REM sleep. REM is essential to awakening feeling rested and refreshed and is characterized by muscle atonia, cortical activation, and rapid eye movements.[7] The body is essentially paralyzed and unresponsive, but the brain is highly active and vivid dreams occur here. Respirations become irregular, rapid, and shallow, and atonia of the nondiaphragmatic respiratory muscles leads to hypoventilation and a fall in Pao_2 and concomitant rise in $Paco_2$. Heart rate and blood pressure increase. As expected, most arousals occur during NREM when muscle tone is lost and the body is essentially paralyzed.

Normal sleep progresses through NREM stages 1 to 3 in cycles lasting 90 to 110 minutes (4–6 cycles per night), before REM sleep occurs (**Fig. 1**). REM is then followed by more NREM stage 2 sleep, before resuming the progression toward deeper sleep. REM dominates the latter half of sleep with each REM cycle becoming progressively longer as awakening nears.

SLEEP-DISORDERED BREATHING

SDB can be categorized into obstructive sleep apnea (OSA), or patients who "cannot breathe" due to obstruction of the oropharyngeal airway, or central sleep apnea (CSA), or patients who "will not breathe," due to the loss of respiratory drive. Of the two, OSA is the most common form of SDB and affects at least 25 million Americans.[8] In OSA, the thoraco-abdominal muscles continue the effort of breathing, but the movement of

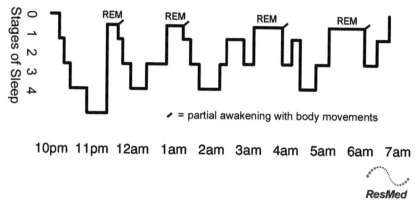

Fig. 1. Stages of sleep. (Copyright © ResMed Limited. All rights reserved.)

air through the upper airway is partially or totally obstructed. Paradoxic movement of the thoraco-abdominal muscles can be seen, as the body struggles to move air against a closed glottis. The effort to breathe continues until the patient is briefly aroused, upper airway muscle tone is restored (usually accompanied by a loud snore), the obstruction is relieved, and effective breathing resumes. The sleeper is likely unaware of this occurrence. A repetitive cyclic pattern of intermittent hypoxia-arousal-reoxygenation results in increased inspiratory effort, sympathetic nerve activity (SNA), negative intrathoracic pressures, and ensuing surges in blood pressure and heart rate.

CSA occurs due to the periodic loss of brainstem-driven respiratory drive. CSA is seen with altitude sickness, narcotic use, or in underlying medical conditions, such as stroke, Parkinson disease, obesity, or HF. Cheyne-Stokes respirations, also known as periodic breathing, is a type of CSA that is characterized by oscillation of tidal volume with crescendo-decrescendo patterns separated by a prolonged apneic event.

The pathophysiology of CSA is complex, as the signal from the brainstem to breathe does not reach the diaphragm and no inspiratory effort is made. This makes $Paco_2$ the only stimulus for respiration during sleep for these patients. As such, any increase in $Paco_2$ will stimulate respiration, whereas a fall in $Paco_2$ below the closely regulated apneic threshold will cause apnea.[9] As previously described, at sleep onset, respirations decrease, and $Paco_2$ increases above the apneic threshold. This chemosensitivity induces hyperventilation that is terminated only when $Paco_2$ declines and the central drive to breathe fades. Respirations are temporarily halted, causing $Paco_2$ to again rise. Once started, this cyclic pattern is self-perpetuating.

CONSEQUENCES OF SLEEP-DISORDERED BREATHING ON HEART FAILURE

Regardless of the type, SDB has many consequences for the cardiovascular system. In addition to SNA, oxidative stress, systemic inflammation, and endothelial dysfunction are seen. Intermittent hypoxemia and hypercapnea decrease oxygen delivery throughout the body, leading to organ dysfunction. SDB has been identified as an independent risk factor for hypertension[10] and is a serious risk factor for other CVD, such as atrial and ventricular arrhythmias,[10,11] stroke,[12,13] coronary artery disease,[10] sudden cardiac death,[11] and HF.[10,14]

In HF, increased systemic vascular resistance, left ventricular work, and wall stress from exaggerated negative intrathoracic pressures, combined with decreased myocardial oxygen delivery, further challenge an already struggling heart. SDB is found in a staggering 47% to 76% of individuals with HF, whether due to HF with reduced ejection fraction (HFrEF) or HF with preserved ejection fraction.[10,15–17] In acute decompensated HF, 75% of hospitalized patients have been found to have SDB.[18] Just like HF, the incidence of SDB increases with age and is associated with worse outcomes, including increased mortality.[19,20] Initially OSA predominates over CSA, but as left ventricular function declines and symptoms worsen, this switches and CSA becomes more prevalent.[21] Yet these at-risk individuals remain largely unrecognized and untreated.

IDENTIFYING PATIENTS WITH SLEEP-DISORDERED BREATHING

Because of the high prevalence of SDB in the HF population, routine screening is necessary for early identification and treatment. This is especially important for patients with frequent rehospitalizations. A thorough history is required to differentiate between symptoms of HF and SDB. However, this is challenging, as the conditions have some overlapping symptoms, such as sleepiness and fatigue. A patient's sleep partner may provide information on snoring, witnessed apneic events, irregular breathing, or nocturnal dyspnea,[22,23] but not all patients have these typical symptoms, reinforcing the need to actively seek SDB in all patients with HF.[24] Although several sleep-screening tools are available, such as the Berlin Questionnaire or the Pittsburgh Sleep Quality Index, none have been validated in patients with HF, making patient identification more challenging.[25]

In a large outpatient registry of more than 6800 stable patients with HF, left ventricular ejection fraction less than 25%, male gender, older age, increased body mass index ($\geq$30 kg/m^2), atrial fibrillation, and New York Heart Association (NYHA) III/IV symptoms were shown to be clinical predictors of sleep apnea.[26] This suggests that the presence of one or more of the predictors should prompt clinicians to suspect SDB. Initially used by anesthesia to determine intubation difficulties, determining the patient's Mallampati score, based on tonsil size and size of the oral space, may be helpful in identifying those more likely to have OSA.[8,23]

A higher prevalence and severity of CSA is noted in patients with HF who are older, male, and have a history of atrial fibrillation. More severe HF indicators, such as low ejection fraction, elevated B-type natriuretic peptides, and increased right heart pressures, are also noted with CSA, which should be included in the list of differential diagnoses.[24]

The gold standard for evaluating sleep and diagnosing sleep disorders is polysomnography (PSG). Most commonly done as an outpatient, many biophysical parameters are assessed during PSG, including airflow, abdominal-thoracic movement, electrocardiogram, electrooculogram, electroencephalography, pulse oximetry, skeletal muscle movement, and behavioral aspects, such as body position or movements[27] (**Fig. 2**).

Box 1 lists the terms to report PSG results. Of importance is the Apnea-Hypopnea Index (AHI), a measurement used primarily to diagnose OSA. The AHI is computed by adding the total number of apneic or hypopneic events divided by the total hours of sleep, and a normal AHI is 5 or less per hour. The threshold used to diagnose OSA and initiate treatment is an AHI of 15 or more per hour, meaning essentially that the patient has 15 or more significant respiratory events every hour of sleep (**Fig. 3**). Severe OSA occurs when the AHI is 30 or more, but it is not unusual to see AHIs in the 100s or more. It is no wonder these patients complain of constant fatigue.[24]

TREATMENT OF SLEEP-DISORDERED BREATHING IN HEART FAILURE

Regardless of the type of SDB, optimization of all indicated HF therapies is critical for improved patient outcomes. This includes diuretics for volume and symptom management, angiotensin-converting enzyme inhibitors or angiotensin receptor blockers to

A

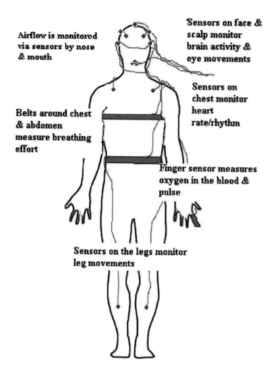

Airflow is monitored via sensors by nose & mouth

Sensors on face & scalp monitor brain activity & eye movements

Sensors on chest monitor heart rate/rhythm

Belts around chest & abdomen measure breathing effort

Finger sensor measures oxygen in the blood & pulse

Sensors on the legs monitor leg movements

B

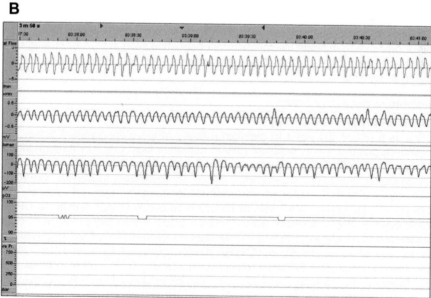

Fig. 2. (*A, B*) PSG. (*C*) PSG showing OSA. (Copyright © ResMed Limited. All rights reserved.)

C

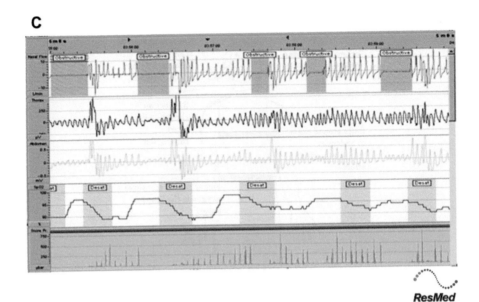

ResMed

Fig. 2. (continued).

block the renin-angiotensin-aldosterone system, and beta-blockers to diminish the effects of SNA.[28] However, it is not unreasonable to think therapeutic efficacy of these medications is obviated by the nightly and repeated neurohormonal surges seen with SDB.

Treatment of SDB primarily consists of noninvasive ventilatory support devices that deliver pressure to mitigate the mechanical obstruction seen in OSA or strategies to stabilize gas exchange in CSA. These pressure devices and other options are discussed as follows.

Noninvasive Ventilatory Support

Positive airway pressure therapy

Acting as a pneumatic splint to maintain patency of the oropharyngeal airway, the continuous positive airway pressure (CPAP) delivers a fixed pressure throughout the respiratory cycle.[29–31] The benefits of CPAP have been extensively studied and include improvements in cardiac performance,[31–33] respiratory function and oxygenation improvements,[30] reduced readmission rates, and improved clinical outcomes.[6,19,34] However, CPAP fails to reduce mortality in CSA.[12] Similar to CPAP, bilevel positive airway pressure (BiPAP) uses a higher inspiratory pressure to open the airway and a lower expiratory pressure. Several small studies of BiPAP in patients with HF have shown improvement of NYHA classifications and decreased AHI.[35] However, there is insufficient evidence to support BiPAP use in HF except in those who have failed CPAP, and other therapies discussed later in this article.[35] Rather than using a fixed pressure, autotitrating CPAP (autoPAP) provides variable pressures to maintain airway patency and decrease that pressure if no abnormal respiratory events are detected. AutoPAP devices also can be programmed to CPAP and BiPAP modes as necessary. Regardless of the device, the goal is to adjust pressures so that the AHI is reduced and the patient has improvements in sleep and other symptoms of sleep deprivation and SDB.

Box 1
Definitions of common sleep respiratory parameters

Apnea

Cessation of respiration for at least 10 seconds. Reduction in airflow by at least 80%

Arousal

Disruption from sleep that lasts from 3 to 15 seconds; refers to a change from a deeper stage to a lighter stage of non–rapid eye movement sleep

Awakening

An arousal from sleep that lasts more than 15 seconds; may be remembered by the sleeper

Hypopnea

Reduction in thoraco-abdominal movement or airflow by 50% to 80% for at least 10 seconds with at least a 4% reduction in oxygen saturation from pre-event values OR at least 3% or greater oxygen desaturation from pre-event associated with an arousal

Apnea-Hypopnea Index (AHI)

Total number of apneic or hypopneic events divided by the total hours of sleep. Classified as follows:

    None/minimal: AHI <5 per hour

    Mild: AHI ≥5, but <15 per hour

    Moderate: AHI ≥15, but <30 per hour

    Severe: AHI ≥30 per hour

Desaturation

Defined as a decline in peripheral pulse oximetry (normal saturation is 95%). Classified as follows:

    Mild: desaturation to 86%

    Moderate: 80%–85%

    Severe: 79% or less

Adaptive servo-ventilation therapy

Adaptive servo-ventilation (ASV) devices have a built-in servocontroller allowing for automatic adjustments of pressure on a breath-by-breath basis to maintain steady minute ventilation. In studies comparing the effects of oxygen, CPAP, BiPAP, and ASV on central events and sleep quality, ASV was most effective in reducing respiratory events.[36,37] A meta-analysis of ASV showed improvement in cardiac performance and decreased AHI in conjunction with improved adherence, as compared with CPAP.[35] However, a prospective trial in HFrEF was halted due to increased relative cardiovascular mortality rate for those receiving ASV.[36]

In those with CSA, the goal is to prevent hypocapnea and break the periodic breathing cycle. With sensors that detect central apneas and respond by delivering breaths at prescribed volume and rates to match the patient's baseline minute ventilation, ASV better regulates airflow and may be better tolerated by the patient.[9]

Supplemental Oxygen

Research has shown the nocturnal use of oxygen in CSA does not offer outcome benefits over CPAP or ASV.[9] Unlike CPAP or ASV, oxygen alone does not alleviate any upper airway obstruction that accompanies CSA, nor will oxygenation be enhanced in

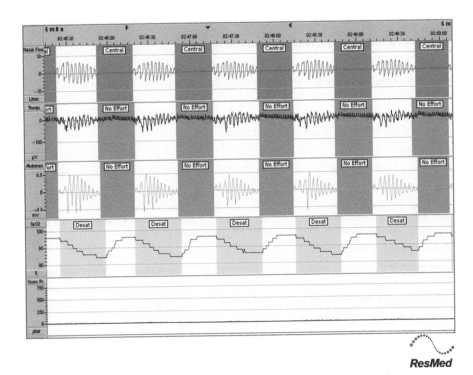

Fig. 3. PSG showing CSA. (Copyright © ResMed Limited. All rights reserved.)

the absence of respiration. However, oxygen may be of best use in patients who cannot tolerate pressure support therapies.

Administration of nocturnal carbon dioxide to prevent hypocapnea has been explored as a potential treatment of CSA, but it is difficult to deliver in an outpatient setting and may increase SNA.[9] Therefore, it is not currently recommended.

Cardiac Pacing

By increasing the intrinsic atrial rate and subsequently increasing cardiac output, atrial overdrive pacing has been evaluated in several small studies of patients with CSA. However, results have been incongruent, with some studies showing reduced CSA events and another showing no effect.[9]

In patients indicated for cardiac resynchronization therapy (CRT) and who have CSA, CRT has been shown to reduce CSA events[38] and improve sleep quality.[39] However, further research is needed to better determine the efficacy of CRT in this subset of patients with HF.

Pharmacologic Interventions

Acetazolamide, a mild diuretic that produces metabolic acidosis, has been studied in CSA. By decreasing $Paco_2$, acetazolamide increases the apneic threshold and reduces respiratory events and improves nocturnal oxygen desaturations. However, acetazolamide can lead to hypokalemia, due to urinary excretion of potassium, and increased likelihood of arrhythmia. Trials of acetazolamide in patients with HF and CSA are necessary to evaluate its safety and efficacy.

A single study of theophylline, a cardiac and respiratory stimulant, in patients with stable HF with CSA showed it reduced apneic events and improved oxygen saturation.[40] Due to its cardiac stimulant and arrhythmogenic effects, further studies are warranted to evaluate its efficacy and safety.

Miscellaneous

Oral sleep appliances

There are many different oral appliances available to assist with oropharyngeal patency. Mandibular repositioning dental devices look like retainers and keep the lower jaw and tongue from compromising the airway. Tongue-retaining appliances are self-explanatory. Both are most effective in mild to moderate OSA but also may be used in patients with severe OSA who cannot tolerate or will not wear CPAP. Additionally these appliances can be used in complicated OSA cases in conjunction with CPAP. In the United States, only a physician can prescribe the appliance, and fitting must be done by a dentist, oral surgeon, or ear nose and throat physician who has sleep medicine experience.[41]

Phrenic nerve stimulation

Using an implanted, lead-based system to stimulate the phrenic nerve transvenously, phrenic nerve stimulation is under investigation for CSA. This device automatically initiates and terminates therapy as needed. In a multicenter, international study there was a 56% decrease in AHI and favorable effects on sleepiness.[42] Ongoing research on the safety and efficacy of phrenic nerve stimulation is ongoing.

CLINICAL IMPLICATIONS

SDB is quite common in patients with CVD and frequently masquerades as symptoms of HF. Simply asking patients about their sleep quality will likely have a low yield in this population. Therefore, clinicians must be knowledgeable about sleep apnea and its clinical consequences and actively include SDB in their differential diagnoses. Although the optimal strategy to best identify SDB in patients with HF is currently unknown, concerted and consistent efforts to support early identification, diagnosis, and subsequent treatment should be strongly encouraged. Following are some suggestions for accomplishing this:

- Screen all patients with HF for SDB due to a prevalence ranging from 50% to 80%.
  - Obtain a thorough family history, physical examination, and sleep history.
  - Current sleep questionnaires have not been validated in HF.
  - Delayed diagnosis and treatment increases morbidity and mortality for patients with HF.[19,43]
  - Optimize all indicated evidence-based therapies for managing HF.
  - Strongly suspect OSA in patients with left ventricular ejection fraction less than 25%, male gender, older age, increased body mass index ($\geq$30 kg/m^2), atrial fibrillation, and NYHA III/IV symptoms.[26]
- Confirm the diagnosis of SDB.
  - PSG as the "gold standard" for diagnosing SDB.
    - Possible barriers: cost, access to testing centers, scheduling delays, inconvenience of being away from home.
  - Home sleep testing devices are approved and available for use in patients with HF in acute care facilities or at home.[44]
- CPAP is the preferred treatment for OSA.

○ CPAP is effective for both acute and chronic treatment.
  ■ Patients with decompensated HF presenting to the emergency department in acute respiratory distress have better outcomes when noninvasive ventilatory support treatment is not delayed.[30]
○ Home CPAP therapy should be continued during hospitalizations.
○ Assess and facilitate CPAP therapy adherence.
  ■ It requires significant lifestyle and behavioral commitment.
  ■ For patients who are unable to tolerate a full face mask, multiple device-face options are available.
○ Evaluation and treatment initiated during hospitalization has been demonstrated effective in reducing readmission rates and mortality outcomes.[6]
• Additional therapies may be considered when a patient is unable to tolerate CPAP or when CSA is present.

SUMMARY

Early recognition and prompt treatment of SDB has the potential to reduce health care expenses and mitigate the development and progression of CVD. As the front line in patient care, nurses are the obvious choice to lead this charge. Start by simply asking the question "Have you been screened or treated for sleep-disordered breathing?" Regardless of practice setting, starting the conversation is the first step in identification and treatment. Optimization of guideline-directed medical therapy and concurrent treatment of SDB are necessary to improve outcomes in this complex patient population.[28]

REFERENCES

1. Centers for Disease Control and Prevention. Available at: http://www.cdc.gov/features/dssleep/. Accessed May 10, 2015.
2. National Sleep Foundation. Available at: http://sleepfoundation.org/sleep-polls-data/2014-sleep-the-modern-family. Accessed May 10, 2015.
3. Schoenborn CA, Adams PF. Health behaviors of adults: United States, 2005–2007. National Center for Health Statistics. Vital Health Stat 10 2010;10(245):1–132.
4. Institute of Medicine. Sleep disorders and sleep deprivation: an unmet public health problem. Washington, DC: The National Academies Press; 2006.
5. Stopford E, Ravi K, Nayar V. The association of sleep disordered breathing with heart failure and other cardiovascular conditions. Cardiol Res Pract 2013;2013: 356280.
6. Peppard PE, Young T, Barnet JH, et al. Increased prevalence of sleep-disordered breathing in adults. Am J Epidemiol 2013;177(9):1006–14.
7. Stevens MS. Normal sleep, sleep physiology and sleep deprivation. 2013. Available at: http://emedicine.medscape.com/article/1188226-overview. Accessed May 10, 2015.
8. Adult Obstructive Sleep Apnea Task Force of the American Academy of Sleep Medicine. Clinical guideline for the evaluation, management and long-term care of obstructive sleep apnea in adults. J Clin Sleep Med 2009;5(3):263–76.
9. Costanzo MR, Khayat R, Ponikowski P, et al. Mechanisms and clinical consequences of untreated central sleep apnea in heart failure. J Am Coll Cardiol 2015;65(1):72–84.
10. Benjamin JA, Lewis KE. Sleep-disordered breathing and cardiovascular disease. Postgrad Med J 2008;84:15–22.
11. Gami AS, Pressman G, Caples SM, et al. Association of atrial fibrillation and obstructive sleep apnea. Circulation 2004;110(4):364–7.

12. Yaggi HK, Concato J, Kernan WN, et al. Obstructive sleep apnea as a risk factor for stroke and death. N Engl J Med 2005;353(19):2034–41.

13. Dyken ME, Somers VK, Yamada T, et al. Investigating the relationship between stroke and obstructive sleep apnea. Stroke 1996;27:401–7.

14. Bradley T, Logan A, Kimoff R, et al. Continuous positive airway pressure for central sleep apnea and heart failure. N Engl J Med 2005;353:2025–33.

15. Bitter T, Westerheide N, Faber L, et al. Adaptive servoventilation in diastolic heart failure and Cheyne–Stokes respiration. Eur Respir J 2010;36:385–92.

16. Vazir A, Hastings PC, Dayer M, et al. A high prevalence of sleep disordered breathing in men with mild symptomatic chronic heart failure due to left ventricular systolic dysfunction. Eur J Heart Fail 2007;9:243–50.

17. Javaheri J. Sleep disorders in systolic heart failure: a prospective study of 100 male patients. Int J Cardiol 2006;106:21–8.

18. Khayat RN, Jarjoura D, Patt B, et al. In-hospital testing for sleep disordered breathing in hospitalized patients with decompensated heart failure: report of prevalence and patient characteristics. J Card Fail 2009;9(15):739–46.

19. Khayat R, Jarjoura D, Porter K, et al. Sleep disordered breathing and post-discharge mortality in patients with acute heart failure. Eur Heart J 2015;36(23):1463–9.

20. Wang H, Parker JD, Newton GE, et al. Influence of obstructive sleep apnea on mortality in patients with heart failure. J Am Coll Cardiol 2007;49:1625–31.

21. Oldenburg O. Cheyne-Stokes respiration in chronic heart failure—treatment with adaptive servoventilation therapy. Circ J 2012;76(10):2305–17.

22. Somers VK, White DP, Amin R, et al. Sleep apnea and cardiovascular disease: an American Heart Association/American Heart Association Council for High Blood Pressure Research Professional Education Committee, Council on Clinical Cardiology, Stroke Council, and Council on Cardiovascular Nursing. J Am Coll Cardiol 2008;52:686–717.

23. Khayat R, Small R, Rathman L, et al. Sleep-disordered breathing in heart failure: identifying and treating an important but often unrecognized comorbidity in heart failure patients. J Card Fail 2013;19(6):431–44.

24. Grimm W, Koehler U. Cardiac arrhythmias and sleep-disordered breathing in patients with heart failure. Int J Mol Sci 2014;15(10):18693–705.

25. Silva GE, Vana KD, Goodwinm JL, et al. Identification of patients with sleep disordered breathing: comparing the four-variable screening tool, STOP, STOP-Bang, and Epworth Sleepiness scales. J Clin Sleep Med 2011;7(5):467–72.

26. Woehrle H, Arzt M, Oldenburg O, et al. Prevalence and predictors of sleep-disordered breathing in patients with stable chronic heart failure: final data of the SCHLA-HF Registry. J Am Coll Cardiol 2015;65(10_S).

27. Iber C, Ancoli-Israel S, Chesson AL, et al. The AASM manual for the scoring of sleep and associated events: rules, terminology and technical specifications. Westchester (IL): American Academy of Sleep Medicine; 2007.

28. Yancy CM, Jessup M, Bozkurt B, et al. 2013 ACCF/AHA guideline for the management of heart failure: executive summary: a report of the American College of Cardiology Foundation/American Heart Association task force on practice guidelines. Circulation 2013;128:1810–52.

29. Burns B. Noninvasive ventilation: a practical guide. Emerg Med 2015;47(1):20.

30. Kato T, Suda S, Kasai T. Positive airway pressure therapy for heart failure. World J Cardiol 2014;6(11):1175–91.

31. Manusukhani M, Kolla BP, Rama K. International classification of sleep disorders 2 and American Academy of Sleep Medicine practice parameters for central sleep apnea. Sleep Med Clin 2014;9:1–11.

32. Mansfield DR, Gollogly NC, Kaye DM, et al. Controlled trial of continuous positive airway pressure in obstructive sleep apnea and heart failure. Am J Respir Crit Care Med 2004;169:361–6.
33. Kaneko Y, Floras J, Phil D, et al. Cardiovascular effects of continuous positive airway pressure in patients with heart failure and obstructive sleep apnea. N Engl J Med 2003;348(13):1233–41.
34. Sharma S, Gupta A, Rubin S, et al. Treatment of sleep disordered breathing in patients admitted for decompensated heart failure reduces 6 months hospital visits. J Am Coll Cardiol 2015;65(10_S).
35. Aurora R, Chowdhuri S, Ramar K, et al. The treatment of central sleep apnea syndromes in adults: practice parameters with an evidence-based literature review and meta-analyses. Sleep 2013;35(1):17–40.
36. ResMed. Available at: http://www.resmed.com/content/dam/resmed/global/documents/serve-hf/Healthcare_Professionals_SERVE-HF_FAQs.pdf. Accessed May 14, 2015.
37. Skobel EC, Sinha AM, Norra C, et al. Effect of cardiac resynchronization therapy on sleep quality, quality of life, and symptomatic depression in patients with chronic heart failure and Cheyne– Stokes respiration. Sleep Breath 2005;9: 159–66.
38. Kasai T, Narui K, Dohi T, et al. First experience of using new adaptive servo-ventilation device for Cheyne–Stokes respiration with central sleep apnea among Japanese patients with congestive heart failure. Circ J 2006;70:1148–54.
39. Sinha AM, Skobel EC, Breithardt OA, et al. Cardiac resynchronization therapy improves central sleep apnea and Cheyne-Stokes respiration in patients with chronic heart failure. J Am Coll Cardiol 2004;44:68–71.
40. Javaheri S, Parker TJ, Wexler L, et al. Effect of theophylline on sleep-disordered breathing in heart failure. N Engl J Med 1996;335:562–7.
41. Conley RS. Management of sleep apnea: a critical look at intra-oral appliances. Orthod Craniofac Res 2015;18(Suppl 1):83–90.
42. Abraham WT, Oldenburg O, Jagielski D, et al. The long term effects of the Remede system in the treatment of central sleep apnea. Paper presented at: European Society of Cardiology – Heart Failure 2014. Athens (Greece), May 19, 2014.
43. Nakamura S, Asai K, Kubota Y, et al. Impact of sleep-disordered breathing and efficacy of positive airway pressure on mortality in patients with chronic heart failure and sleep-disordered breathing: a meta-analysis. Clin Res Cardiol 2015; 104(3):208–16.
44. Qaseem A, Dallas P, Owens DK, et al. Diagnosis of obstructive sleep apnea in adults: a clinical practice guideline from the American College of Physicians: diagnosis of obstructive sleep apnea in adults. Ann Intern Med 2014;161(3): 210–20.

Patient Safety Coalition

A Focus on Heart Failure

Jennifer Kitchens, MSN, RN, ACNS-BC, CVRN[a],*, Joanna Kingery, PharmD[b],
James H. Fuller, PharmD[c], Arif Nazir, MD[d]

KEYWORDS

- Hospitals • Skilled nursing facilities • Home care • Interdisciplinary collaboration
- Heart failure readmissions • Population health • Post-acute care

---

KEY POINTS

- Heart failure (HF) readmissions are costly and may indicate gaps in care.
- Developing a regional patient safety coalition is one strategy to address HF readmission rates.
- It is important to include skilled nursing facilities and home health care agencies in brainstorming for sustainable solutions to reduce HF-related readmissions.

INTRODUCTION

Heart failure (HF) is a significant health care issue. Approximately 5.7 million Americans have HF, with 870,000 new cases being diagnosed each year.[1] HF is reported to be the cause in 1 out of 9 deaths.[1] In 2011, there were 284,388 deaths for HF any-mention mortality, and HF was the underlying cause of 58,309 of these deaths.[1] The total cost for HF in 2012 was approximately $30.7 billion, and 68% of this was direct medical costs.[2] The cost of HF will continue to increase. The total cost of HF is projected to increase an estimated 127% to $69.7 billion from 2012 to the year 2030.[2] From 2012 to 2030, the prevalence of HF is projected to increase 46%, leading to more than 8 million adults older than 18 years with HF.[2]

   HF patient readmissions result in escalated health care costs and indicate poor patient management and gaps in care. These gaps represent a significant patient safety

---

The authors declare they have no conflicts of interest.
[a] Acuity Adaptable, Eskenazi Health, 720 Eskenazi Avenue, Indianapolis, IN 46202, USA;
[b] Statewide Advanced Heart Care, Indiana University Health, 1707 Senate Boulevard, Indianapolis, IN 46202, USA; [c] Indianapolis Coalition for Patient Safety, Inc, 351 West 10th Street, Suite 342, Indianapolis, IN 46202, USA; [d] Eskenazi Health, 720 Eskenazi Avenue, Indianapolis, IN 46202, USA
* Corresponding author.
E-mail address: jennifer.kitchens@eskenazihealth.edu

issue and can negatively affect patient outcomes. Among Medicare beneficiaries, all-cause readmissions within 30 days following HF hospitalization approaches 25% nationally.[3] One strategy to reduce readmission rates in patients with HF is to collaborate through a patient safety coalition. This article describes how the Indianapolis Coalition for Patient Safety (ICPS) addressed the issue of hospital readmissions for patients diagnosed with HF.

BACKGROUND OF PATIENT SAFETY COALITIONS

In several states, private and public health care providers, purchasers, consumers, and regulators have recognized the value of coordinating their efforts to create an environment that enhances safety. Regional public/private patient safety coalitions have been formed in several states.[4] Patient safety coalitions typically have diverse membership, often including real or potential competitors within the group.[4] They voluntarily come together to address the common goal of reducing the harm that comes to patients, professionals, and institutions when a medical error or an adverse event occurs.[4] By using evidence-based strategies and process improvement projects, regional patient safety coalitions have shown a reduction in 30-day readmission rates of patients diagnosed with HF.[5]

The Indiana Hospital Association (IHA) has created 11 regional patient safety coalitions (including ICPS) that blanket the state geographically.[6] These patient safety coalitions are made up of dedicated professionals, including hospital leadership, doctors, pharmacists, and nurses, who collaborate to improve patient safety[6] **(Fig. 1)**.

The ICPS provides a forum for Indianapolis-area hospitals to share best practices and work together to solve patient safety issues.[7] A free-standing nonprofit organization, the ICPS Board is composed of chief executive officers and representatives from medical, nursing, quality/safety, and pharmacy from the 6 major health systems located in Indianapolis: Community Health Network, Eskenazi Health, Franciscan-St. Francis Health, Indiana University Health, Richard L. Roudebush Veterans Affairs Medical Center, and St. Vincent Health.[7] Although competitors in the market place, hospital leaders came together and agreed to not compete on safety. Coalition hospitals pool their expert resources to accelerate patient safety improvements through community-wide efforts.[7] In addition, ICPS[7] works closely with many community partners, including IHA,[8] Marion County Department of Public Health, schools of medicine, nursing, and pharmacy to name a few.

The ICPS historically achieved accelerated outcomes by sharing resources, evidence-based best practices, performance targets, accountability, and learning. ICPS members undertake projects that focus on patient-centered strategies to improve safety and patient outcomes. Pulling content experts from each of the health systems and community partners, ICPS has formed initiative-specific work groups addressing patient safety issues in medication safety, perioperative safety, blood safety, pediatrics, use of contrast media, workplace violence, multidrug-resistant organisms, and reducing HF readmissions.[8] Simply stated ICPS' mission is to provide a forum for Indianapolis-area hospitals to share information about best practices and work together to solve patient safety issues in Indianapolis and surrounding county hospitals.[8]

The ICPS Targeting Prevention of Heart Failure Patient Hospital Readmissions within 30 Days following Hospital Discharge work group was formed in 2009 with

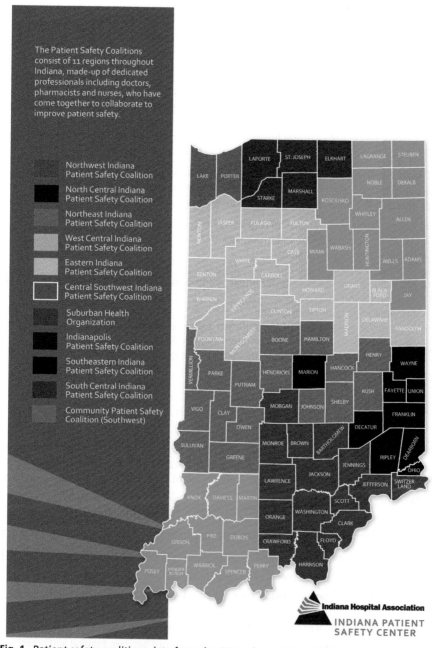

The Patient Safety Coalitions consist of 11 regions throughout Indiana, made-up of dedicated professionals including doctors, pharmacists and nurses, who have come together to collaborate to improve patient safety.

Northwest Indiana Patient Safety Coalition

North Central Indiana Patient Safety Coalition

Northeast Indiana Patient Safety Coalition

West Central Indiana Patient Safety Coalition

Eastern Indiana Patient Safety Coalition

Central Southwest Indiana Patient Safety Coalition

Suburban Health Organization

Indianapolis Patient Safety Coalition

Southeastern Indiana Patient Safety Coalition

South Central Indiana Patient Safety Coalition

Community Patient Safety Coalition (Southwest)

Indiana Hospital Association
INDIANA PATIENT SAFETY CENTER

Fig. 1. Patient safety coalitions data from the IHA Indiana Patient Safety Center. The Patient Safety Coalitions consist of 11 regions throughout Indiana, made-up of dedicated professionals including doctors, pharmacists and nurses, who have come together to collaborate to improve patient safety. (*Courtesy of* Indiana Hospital Association, Indianapolis, IN; with permission. Available at: http://www.ihaconnect.org/Indiana-Hospitals/Pages/Regional-Patient-Safety-Coalitions-Map.aspx?PrintPreview#. Accessed May 28, 2015.)

representatives from all 6 health systems. Over the next 5 years, work was completed in 4 primary focuses:

- Coalition consensus on implementable tactics to improve preventable HF patient readmissions
- Collaborating with Central Indiana skilled nursing facilities (SNFs) on minimum care standards for treatment of patients with HF
- Improving verbal handoff communication for patients transferred from hospitals to SNFs
- Collaborating with Central Indiana home health care agencies on minimum care standards for treatment of patients with HF in home health care agencies

The 2013 American College of Cardiology Foundation/American Heart Association's guidelines for the management of HF describe following common factors that may precipitate HF admissions and readmissions[9]:

- Nonadherence with medical regimen and sodium or fluid restriction
- Acute myocardial ischemia/infarction
- Uncorrected hypertension
- Valvular disease
- Atrial fibrillation, cardiac arrhythmias, ventricular tachycardia, bradycardia, conduction abnormalities
- Adverse effects of medications
- Initiation of medications that increase salt retention (eg, steroids, thiazolidinediones, nonsteroidal antiinflammatory medications)
- Recent addition of negative inotropic medications (eg, verapamil, nifedipine, diltiazem, beta-blockers)
- Pulmonary embolism
- Excessive alcohol or illicit drug use
- Endocrine abnormalities (eg, diabetes, thyroid disorders)
- Concurrent or systemic infections

The work group identified a need for each member hospital to perform a self-assessment for the root causes of HF related readmissions to their hospital systems. After reviewing the hospital self-assessments, eight root causes of HF readmissions emerged (**Box 1**).

Box 1
Root causes of HF readmissions identified through self-assessment

Lack of timely access to outpatient follow-up after discharge from the hospital

Failure of proper medications handoff between providers and across sites of care during transitions

Lack of care coordination or ownership across sites of care

Accountability for patients after discharge is not well defined between hospital and other providers.

Lack of assigned or designated personnel for scheduling follow-up appointments

Lack of HF clinic resources

Lack of standardized processes to assess patient risk for readmission

Patients inability to navigate the healthcare system

TACTICS TO REDUCE READMISSION RATES

The Case Management Society of America convened the National Transitions of Care Coalition (NTOCC) to develop recommendations on actions that all participants in the health care delivery system can take to improve the quality of care transitions, including the development of policies, tools, resources, and recommend actions and protocols to guide and support providers and patients in achieving safe and effective transitions of care.[10]

The NTOCC work group identified the following key elements of optimal transitions of care[9]:

- Accountable provider at all points of care transition
- An updated and proactive patient care plan including advance directives
- Medication reconciliation
- Admission and discharge planning
- Follow-up appointment tracking
- End-of-life decision making
- Adequate and accurate (transfer) communication between providers and care settings
- Patient and family education

Hospital-To-Home (H2H) is a national quality-improvement campaign of the American College of Cardiology and Institute for Healthcare Improvement.[11] The H2H initiative is a resource for hospitals and cardiovascular care providers committed to improving transitions from hospital to home and reducing their risk of federal penalties associated with high readmission rates.[11] The H2H initiative outlined three process improvement projects[11]:

- See you in Seven: The goal is for all patients discharged with a diagnosis of HF to have a follow-up appointment scheduled within 7 days of hospital discharge.
- Mind your Meds: The goal is for clinicians and patients discharged with a diagnosis of HF to work together and ensure optimal medication management.
- Signs and Symptoms: The goal is to activate patients to recognize early warning signs and have a plan to address them.[11]

Based on these projects, the ICPS Targeting Prevention of Heart Failure Patient Hospital Readmissions within 30 Days following Hospital Discharge work group members reached consensus on 4 key tactics to improve preventable HF patient readmissions:

- Assure that patients have access to their medications and are knowledgeable about the medications.
- Early follow-up: Patients have a follow-up appointment scheduled within a week of discharge and are able to get there.
- Symptom management: Patients fully comprehend the signs and symptoms that require medical attention and know who to contact should they occur.
- Care management after discharge: Patients are evaluated for home health care referral.

TRANSITIONS OF CARE: HOSPITAL TO SKILLED NURSING FACILITIES

In patients with HF, transitions of care typically refer to individual interventions and programs with multiple bundled activities that are designed to improve shifts or transitions from one setting to the next.[12] Most often, these interventions are focused on transitions from hospital to home.[12,13] There is a gap in the literature related to transitions from hospital to SNF, and little is known about interventions to reduce hospitalization of patients with HF who are discharged to post-acute care settings, specifically SNF.[13] However, one SNF designed a skilled heart unit program that resulted in better HF care.[14]

The proportions of 30-day HF readmissions are greater among patients discharged to a SNF compared with patients discharged to home (27% vs 21%, $P = .031$). After adjustment for age and sex, patients discharged to an SNF had a 40% increase in the odds of having hospital readmissions within 30 days after HF compared with those discharged to home.[15] Characteristics most associated with patients with HF admitted to an SNF were longer lengths of hospital stay, older age, history of depression or stroke, and female sex.[16] For ICPS member hospitals, 2010 baseline data provided by the IHA showed that there was a 20.2% readmission rate for patients with HF for any reason from an SNF.

After identifying the need to collaborate with post-acute care facilities to improve outcomes, Indianapolis-area SNFs were invited to participate with the ICPS Targeting Prevention of Heart Failure Patient Hospital Readmissions within 30 Days following Hospital Discharge work group to improve care and care transitions for patients with HF in these post-acute care facilities. The ICPS Targeting Prevention of Heart Failure Patient Hospital Readmissions within 30 Days following Hospital Discharge work group expanded in 2011 to include SNF representatives to address care transitions of patients with HF discharged from hospitals to SNFs. Local SNFs embraced the opportunity to collaborate to reduce readmissions. In 2011, data provided by the IHA showed ICPS hospitals there was a 16.7% readmission rate for patients with HF for any reason from an SNF.

A retrospective review of bundled interventions for enhancing transitions of (care) heart failure patients that included weight monitoring, sodium restriction, medication review and reconciliation, importance of follow-up appointments, and education showed that these interventions led to better outcomes.[12] The ICPS work group reached consensus on 6 minimum standards of care for SNFs to provide better HF care that were then also endorsed by Indiana Society of Post-acute and Long-term Care Medicine (IMDA).[17] Refer to **Table 2**, Minimum SNF standards for the care of patients with HF. These standards were intended to be practical and achievable so that a broad level of SNF participation could be attained but SNFs were also encouraged to take initiatives beyond these minimum standards.

IMPLEMENTATION OF MINIMUM CARE STANDARDS FOR THE CARE OF PATIENTS WITH HEART FAILURE

The ICPS Targeting Prevention of Heart Failure Patient Hospital Readmissions within 30 Days following Hospital Discharge work group agreed that ICPS leaders should send a letter to SNF administrators to explain the initiative and invite their organization's full participation. The letter became the tool used to facilitate discussions between hospitals and their SNF partners. Work group members provided an educational session to SNF leadership to further educate and gain buy-in from SNF. Individual SNFs were further incentivized to participate because of the opportunity to be recognized by ICPS as committing to these minimum care standards and the potential to improve relationships with local health systems. Nearly 80 facilities signed letters of commitment to adopt the standards and implement them as protocol for their HF residents. The coalition posted a list of them online, where case managers could access it.

In 2015, the initial work with SNFs was revisited with revised minimum SNF standards (**Table 1**).

Table 1
Minimum SNF standards for the care of patients with HF

Year 2011	Year 2015
1. Use best practices in transition of patients with HF: a. Medication reconciliation (focus on diuretic, beta-blocker, ACE-inhibitor and antiplatelet therapy) b. Discharge summary available in the chart within 72 h of admission c. Clarification of code status within 24 h of admission d. Initial plan of care goals within 72 h of admission	1. Use best practices in transition of patients with HF: a. Perform medication reconciliation (focus on diuretic, beta-blocker, ACE inhibitor, and antiplatelet therapy) at the time of admission. b. Make all efforts to have the discharge summary available in the chart within 72 h of admission. c. Clarify patient advance care plans and code status within 24 h of admission and, when applicable, complete the POST[a] form within a reasonable time frame. d. Establish initial plan of care goals within 2 h of admission.
2. Availability of a low-salt diet (2 g/d)	2. Assure availability of a low-salt diet (2 g/d).
3. Daily weights for 30 d and then 3 times per wk thereafter	3. Perform daily weights for 30 d and then 3 times per wk thereafter.
4. Initial provider visit within 48 h of admission and at least weekly follow-up visits	4. Facilitate the initial provider visit within 48 h of admission and at least weekly follow-up visits thereafter.
5. Activity as tolerated outside of therapy	5. Promote activity as tolerated outside of therapy.
6. Identification of an HF champion within the facility who leads the quality-improvement efforts for enhanced HF care and implements systems for patient and family education	6. Identify an HF champion within the facility who will assure systems are in place to a. Provide HF education for patients and families in the facility b. Provide HF education to the facility nursing and other staff members c. Train the staff for the use of valid communication tools (eg, STOP and Watch and Situation Background Assessment Recommendation available at www.interact2.net and The Society of Post-acute and Long-term Care Medicine (AMDA) Know-It-ALL series available at www.amda.com) to improve early recognition and communication of HF symptoms to prevent unnecessary hospitalization of patients with HF. d. Continually review quality-improvement efforts for enhanced HF care.

Abbreviations: ACE, angiotensin-converting enzyme; POST, Physician Orders for Scope of Treatment.

[a] The Indiana Physician Orders for Scope of Treatment (POST) form is a new advance care planning tool that helps ensure treatment preferences are honored. It is designed for patients with serious illness.[18,19]

Data from Refs.[10,12,13]

Again, ICPS leaders sent a similar letter inviting SNFs to participate and join in committing to these minimum standards. Key changes included

- Inclusion of systems to clarify advance care plans in addition to code status
- Inclusion of Indiana Physician Orders for Scope of Treatment form[18]
- Delineation of the role of an HF champion

BETTER VERBAL COMMUNICATION

The provision of quality nursing care depends on the handover process. Miscommunication between caregivers may result in delay in treatment, inappropriate treatment, adverse events, omissions of care, increased costs, and inefficiencies from rework.[20] The SNF nurses that joined the ICPS Targeting Prevention of Heart Failure Patient Hospital Readmissions within 30 Days following Hospital Discharge work group reported several patient safety issues regarding verbal handoff communications from hospitals, including no diagnosis with medications (required for SNFs), no diagnosis, incomplete clinical information, lack of current status, lack of recent changes in condition, lack of a plan of care, and no relay of patient-/family-specific concerns. The impact of poor handoff communications included delay in diagnosis or treatment, need for additional testing, potential for falls, and potential transfer back to the hospital.

Although requesting a commitment to the HF care standards fostered ongoing communication and collaboration between the discharging hospital and the admitting facility, in subsequent months the ICPS Targeting Prevention of Heart Failure Patient Hospital Readmissions within 30 Days following Hospital Discharge work group evaluated the potential to standardize verbal transfer information. Because of the complexity and uniqueness of electronic medical records, written/printed transfer information was beyond the scope of this work group.

In order to assess the existing handoff process, the ICPS Targeting Prevention of Heart Failure Patient Hospital Readmissions within 30 Days following Hospital Discharge work group conducted a survey to assess sender and receiver perceptions about the quality of key elements of communication, including timeliness, content of handoff, method, and overall satisfaction. The survey was completed by nursing staff on selected hospital units transferring patients to SNFs and SNF nursing staff in order to collect feedback. Using a Likert scale whereby 5 is strongly agree and 1 is strongly disagree, The ICPS Targeting Prevention of Heart Failure Patient Hospital Readmissions within 30 Days following Hospital Discharge work group agree, the senders (hospitals) rated it a 5 on a 1-to-5 Likert scale; in contrast, the receivers (SNFs) indicated the communication was unclear or incomplete, giving it only a 3 on the same scale. The survey highlighted that there was a disconnect between sending and receiving entities.

The SNF representatives took on the role of developing a tool that pulled pertinent information in a clear, usable way. Initially the work group leaned toward an electronic tool for the handoff, but the wide variation in technologies in use across the area caused them to reconsider. The ICPS Targeting Prevention of Heart Failure Patient Hospital Readmissions within 30 Days following Hospital Discharge work group members agreed that they did not need one more piece of paper. The SNF verbal handoff cue card was born (**Box 2**). The aim was to provide a complete and concise patient report that allowed the accepting nurse to provide care until the written report can be reviewed.

Chief nursing officers at the ICPS member hospitals supported the use of the verbal handoff cue card. Use of the verbal cue card has steadily spread among ICPS participants. Although its impact on HF readmissions is still being measured, early anecdotal reports indicate it has been well received by both senders and receivers. Using the cue

Box 2
SNF verbal handoff cue card

Identifying information

Name

Date of birth

Language

Male/female

Hospital admission date

Current medical information/pertinent information

Admitting diagnosis

Focused patient history

Comorbidities of relevance

Surgery history of relevance

Abnormal laboratory test results or diagnostic test results

Abnormal vital signs

Current weight (bariatric equipment)

Skin issues and treatments with frequency

Current medications

- Review critical medications
- Next time of dosing
- Not including supplements and vitamins

Invasive lines, location, use

Safety precautions (anticipatory concerns)

- Allergies
- Fall risk
- Infection control status

Diet restrictions or feeding precautions

Cognition/behaviors

Code status (Do patients have an out-of-hospital do not resuscitate order?)

Additional family/patient information that may affect transfer or stay

Call back number if there are questions and name of on-coming nurse

Give the receiving staff person the opportunity to ask any questions or clarify information

Send prescriptions for narcotics (if applicable)

card saves time by omitting irrelevant information and streamlines the transfer process.

TRANSITIONS OF CARE: HOSPITAL TO HOME HEALTH CARE

Expanding on the good work and relationship with SNFs, the ICPS Targeting Prevention of Heart Failure Patient Hospital Readmissions within 30 Days following Hospital

Discharge work group began collaborating with the Indiana Association for Home and Hospice Care (IAHHC).[21] The ICPS Targeting Prevention of Heart Failure Patient Hospital Readmissions within 30 Days following Hospital Discharge work group developed minimum HF care standards in 2014 for patients receiving services from home health care agencies (**Box 3**). The standards are considered minimum care standards, and the agencies were encouraged to take initiatives beyond these minimum standards to improve care and reduce the readmissions of patients with HF. The ICPS Targeting Prevention of Heart Failure Patient Hospital Readmissions within 30 Days following Hospital Discharge work group created a letter outlining these minimum standards inviting all home health care agencies in Marion County to participate. By signing the letter, the home health care agencies committed to delivering care at this level and were recognized as such by the ICPS.

The ICPS Targeting Prevention of Heart Failure Patient Hospital Readmissions within 30 Days following Hospital Discharge work group and IAHHC produced an educational webinar for home health care agencies that outlined each standard, discussed the evidence, and gave real-life, practical examples. The webinar aired on September 30, 2014. In total, 110 individuals representing 23 different home health

---

Box 3
2014 home health care minimum standards for patients with HF

1. Start of care/resumption of care completed within 24 hours of hospital discharge

2. Medication reconciliation on admission (focus on diuretic, beta-blocker, ACE inhibitor, and antiplatelet therapy)

3. Initiation of telemonitoring/telehealth for all patients with HF on home health care admission; use of equipment or competent staff for daily monitoring of health metrics (BP, weight, and so forth)

4. Instruction of patients with HF education materials, using teach back method

   a. Instructing and encouraging patients on the recommended low-sodium diet (2 g/d)

   b. Instructing patients on the importance of daily weights, maintenance of recording daily weights, and when/who to call for weight gain

   c. Instructing patients for confidence in the early recognition of HF symptoms and timely actions to resolve the problem and avoid an emergency

5. Instruction, and assistance if appropriate, for scheduling a physician appointment as indicated on discharge instructions; discussion of patients' transportation plans for appointment and encouragement of patients to attend

6. Licensed home health care professional patient visit at least weekly × 4 weeks after hospital discharge

7. Identification of an HF champion within the agency who leads the quality-improvement efforts for enhanced HF care and implements systems for patient and family education regarding HF; must be a licensed health care professional

8. Staff training on HF management and HF patient education

   a. Verification of standardized use of all staff training for all employees on hire and annually thereafter; must use approved training and testing

   b. Verification of standardized nurse training for all licensed nurses on hire and annually thereafter; must use approved training and testing

Abbreviations: ACE, angiotensin-converting enzyme; BP, blood pressure.
   Data from Refs.[9,12,22–28]

care agencies participated in the webinar. In addition, ICPS work group members served as faculty for a panel discussion at the Indiana Association of Home and Hospice Care Annual Conference on May 6, 2015 outlining the same material included in the webinar.

OUTCOMES

From 2010 to 2014, the percentage of HF readmissions for HF has decreased 33%, and ICPS member hospitals have had a 19.2% reduction in HF readmissions for any reason from SNFs (**Table 2**). ICPS recognizes that all of the health systems are also independently working to improve processes and methods to reduce readmissions and does not assert that these improvements are attributed solely to the ICPS Targeting Prevention of Heart Failure Patient Hospital Readmissions within 30 Days following Hospital Discharge work group efforts.

DISCUSSION

The ICPS Targeting Prevention of Heart Failure Patient Hospital Readmissions within 30 Days following Hospital Discharge work group continues to meet regularly, monitors readmission rates, and provides a forum for additional sharing from ICPS members and the authors' SNF and home health care community partners. Work group members feel positive about the potential impact of a project distinctive in its level of collaboration. "By working together, we were able to leverage our size and the scope of what we covered to get the attention of some of our community partners. It is easier to make transformational change once you have a relationship." (Joanna Kingery, PharmD, personal communication, 2015).

SUMMARY

When addressing a complex issue like HF readmissions, there are clear benefits of working with a regional coalition and involving community partners. When forming a regional coalition, do not reinvent the wheel. Use the wealth of experience and knowledge within local entities as well as pulling best practices from evidence-based sources.[4] Because of the complexity of issues and different levels of expertise among providers of care, prioritize the work to be done and work to reach consensus on areas of focus. Coalition meetings should be well organized with clear objectives, agendas, and assignments.[4]

Working with regional coalitions can also present challenges with the potential for conflicting priorities among entities that may otherwise be competitors. A critical element in the success of a coalition is identifying the right blend of stakeholders who bring the necessary talents and resources to achieve identified goals. Building the trust and relationships necessary to create the esprit de corps that comes from working together for a common good may take time.[4]

Table 2 HF readmissions data for ICPS hospitals from IHA					
	2010	2011	2012	2013	2014
HF readmissions for HF (%)	7.37	7.03	5.98	5.33	4.92
HF readmissions for ANY REASON (%)	16.75	15.94	15.03	15.55	13.93
HF readmissions for any reason from SNF (%)	20.20	16.70	16.9	17.58	16.32

ACKNOWLEDGMENTS

The authors would like to acknowledge the ICPS Targeting Prevention of Heart Failure Patient Hospital Readmissions work group members; Indiana Hospital Association; SNFs and home health care agencies who served as key community partners; Indiana Association for Home and Hospice Care; Carol Birk, former President, ICPS; Lisa Sorenson, RN, IU Health, former Chairperson; and the ICPS Targeting Prevention of Heart Failure Patient Hospital Readmissions within 30 Days following Hospital Discharge work group.

REFERENCES

1. Mozaffarian D, Emelia J, Go A, et al. Heart disease and stroke statistics-2015 update: a report from the American Heart Association. Circulation 2015;131:e1–294.
2. Heidenreich PA, Albert NM, Allen LA, et al, On behalf of the American Heart Association Advocacy Coordinating Committee, Council on Arteriosclerosis, Thrombosis and Vascular Biology, Council on Cardiovascular Radiology and Intervention, Council on Clinical Cardiology, Council on Epidemiology and Prevention, and Stroke Council. Forecasting the impact of heart failure in the United States: a policy statement from the American Heart Association. Circ Heart Fail 2013;6:606–60.
3. Krumholz HM, Merrill AR, Schone EM, et al. Patterns of hospital performance in acute myocardial infarction and heart failure 30-day mortality and readmission. Circ Cardiovasc Qual Outcomes 2009;2:407–13.
4. Comden SW, Rosenthal J. Statewide patient safety coalitions: a status report. 2002. Available at: http://www.oregon.gov/OHA/OHPR/HPC/docs/mat04/NASHP Statewide.pdf. Accessed May 28, 2015.
5. Pollard J, Oliver-McNeil S, Patel S, et al. Impact of the development of regional collaborative to reduce 30-day heart failure readmissions. J Nurs Care Qual 2015;30(4):298–305.
6. Indiana Hospital Association. Available at: http://www.ihaconnect.org/Indiana-Hospitals/Pages/Regional-Patient-Safety-Coalitions-Map.aspx?PrintPreview#. Accessed May 28, 2015.
7. Indianapolis Coalition for Patient Safety. Available at: http://www.indypatientsafety.org/. Accessed May 28, 2015.
8. Indianapolis Coalition for Patient Safety Focus Groups. Available at: http://www.indypatientsafety.org/focus_areas.aspx. Accessed May 28, 2015.
9. Yancy CW, Jessup M, Bozkurt B, et al. 2013 ACCF/AHA guideline for the management of heart failure: a report of the American College of Cardiology Foundation/American Heart Association Task Force on Practice Guidelines. Circulation 2013;128:e240–327.
10. National Transitions of Care Coalition (NTOCC). Transitions of care measures paper by the NTOCC. 2008. Available at: http://www.ntocc.org/Portals/0/PDF/Resources/TransitionsOfCare_Measures.pdf. Accessed May 28, 2015.
11. Hospital-To-Home. Available at: http://cvquality.acc.org/Initiatives/H2H.aspx. Accessed May 28, 2015.
12. Albert N, Barnason S, Deswal A, et al. Transitions of care in heart failure: a scientific statement from the American Heart Association. Circ Heart Fail 2015;8:383–409.
13. Pressler SJ. Heart failure patients in skilled nursing facilities: evidence needed. Circ Heart Fail 2011;4:241–3.
14. Nazir A, Dennis ME, Unroe KT. Implementation of a heart failure quality initiative in a skilled nursing facility: lessons learned. J Gerontol Nurs 2014;41(5):26–33.

15. Manemann SM, Chamberlin AM, St. Sauver J. Skilled nursing facilities and 30-day hospital readmissions in heart failure. Circulation 2014;130:A15301.
16. Allen LA, Hernandez AF, Peterson ED. Discharge to a skilled nursing facility and subsequent clinical outcomes among older patients hospitalized for heart failure. Circ Heart Fail 2011;4:293–300.
17. IMDA: Indiana Society of Post-acute and Long-term Care Medicine. Available at: http://www.inmda.com/. Accessed May 28, 2015.
18. Indiana Physician Orders for Scope of Treatment Form (POST). Available at: in. gov/Download.aspx?id=11217. Accessed May 28, 2015.
19. Hickman SE, Keevern E, Hammes BJ. Use of the physician orders for life-sustaining treatment program in the clinical setting: a systematic review of the literature. J Am Geriatr Soc 2015;63(2):341–50.
20. Joint Commission Center for Transforming Healthcare. Handoff Communications Targeted Solutions Tool. Available at: http://www.centerfortransforminghealthcare.org/assets/4/6/HOC_TST_Implementation_Guide.pdf. Accessed May 28, 2015.
21. Indiana Association for Home and Hospice Care (IAHHC). Available at: http://www.iahhc.org/?. Accessed May 28, 2015.
22. Fleming M, Haney T. Improving patient outcomes with better care transition: the role for home health. Cleve Clin J Med 2013;80:eS2–6.
23. Coleman EA, Parry C, Chalmers S, et al. The care transitions intervention: results of a randomized controlled trial. Arch Intern Med 2006;166:1822–8.
24. Inglis S. Structured telephone support or telemonitoring programmes for patients with chronic heart failure. J Evid Based Med 2010;3:228.
25. White M, Garbez R, Brinker CM, et al. Is "teach-back" associated with knowledge retention and hospital readmission in hospitalized heart failure patients? J Cardiovasc Nurs 2013;28(2):137–46.
26. Delaney C, Apostolidis B, Lachapelle L, et al. Home care nurses' knowledge of evidence-based education topics for management of heart failure. Heart Lung 2011;40(4):285–92.
27. Fowler S. Improving community health nurses' knowledge of heart failure education principles: a descriptive study. Home Healthc Nurse 2012;30(2):91–9.
28. Naylor M, Brooten D, Campbell R, et al. Comprehensive discharge planning and home follow-up of hospitalized elders: a randomized clinical trial. JAMA 1999; 281(7):613–20.

The Role of the Nurse Navigator in the Management of the Heart Failure Patient

 CrossMark

Kristin Monza, MSN, RN, CHFN, Dana Harris, BSN, RN, CHFN, Carmen Shaw, MSN, RN-BC*

KEYWORDS

- Nurse navigator • Transitions of care • Self-management • Readmission rates
- Heart-failure

KEY POINTS

- Implementing a nurse navigator has proven to reduce readmission rates among the heart failure patient population.
- HF nurse navigators impact the quality and outcomes of patient care.
- A HF nurse navigator program has been proven to significantly reduce 30-day all-cause hospital readmissions, enhance self-management skills, and improve follow-up compliance.

Webster's dictionary defines a navigator as one who directs the course or the route.[1] The role of the nurse navigator has historically evolved, since the early 1990s, within the field of oncology services and found to be pertinent to the success and care of chronic illness management, providing emotional and educational support as a patient advocate.[2] In 2011, the heart failure (HF) clinic at Carolinas Medical Center (CMC) in Charlotte, North Carolina, decided to implement the position as a new initiative in the care and management of the chronic HF patient population.

A growing portion of the health care budget is spent on delivering care to individuals with a focus on proper patient monitoring and medical management. Annual expenses for HF have been estimated as high as $32 billion in 2013 and this is projected to increase nearly 120% to $70 billion by 2030.[3] Expectations have shifted for the patient to better understand their plan of care, diagnosis and proper self-management skills. HF is a chronic illness that affects more than 5 million patients in the United States and

The authors have no relevant financial or nonfinancial relationships to disclose.
Carolinas Healthcare System, Sanger Heart & Vascular Institute, 1000 Blythe Boulevard, Charlotte, NC 28203, USA
* Corresponding author.
E-mail address: Carmen.Shaw@carolinashealthcare.org

the prevalence is expected to increase by 25% by 2030. The increasing cost burden and adding urgency to the need for consistent care. Much of the cost of HF is attributed to hospital admissions and readmissions.[3] Many readmissions have been linked to variation of care and interventions are aimed at optimizing quality and performance monitoring, medication management, education, and follow-up.[3] Although this population has been known to challenge compliance, a more proactive approach to education, communication, and monitoring can significantly reduce the failure rate as measured by 30-day readmissions (**Table 1**).

As a result of the economic challenges associated with HF, CMC recognized the need to address readmissions. CMC has an Advanced Heart Failure Clinic, which includes a transplant and mechanical circulatory support program and more than 2500 patients, managed under board-certified HF specialists. The hospital has more than 850 HF index admissions each year and HF is among the most common diagnoses across all CHS hospitals. It was recognized that there was significant variation in managing HF across the continuum from primary care through complex inpatient services. An oversight committee was appointed to create a phased plan to improve the quality of care for HF patients. The plan was to include deliverables to decrease unintentional variations in care, identify better ways to manage HF patients across the continuum, and provide appropriate resources and tools for the providers to recognize gaps in care and the management of the HF population. The Rapid Action Change Event team recognized that hospital inpatient quality indicators for HF patients could develop further with the addition of transitional care. As a result of the team's work, in the fourth quarter of 2011, the facility implemented a transitional care clinic, known as the Heart Success Transition Clinic (HSTC). The HSTC was designed to address the potential gap in care between the acute and ambulatory care settings. One of the first roles to implement, design, and expand was the pivotal role of the nurse navigator.

Table 1
Elements of change: where are we going?

Element of Change	Today	Future
Care focus	Sick care	"Health care," wellness, prevention, and disease management
Care management	Manage utilization and cost within a care setting	Manage ongoing health (and optimize care episodes)
Delivery models	Fragmented/silos	Care continuum and coordination (right care, right place, right time)
Care setting	In office/hospital	In home, virtual (e-visits, home monitoring, etc)
Quality measures	Process focused, individual	Outcomes focused, population based
Payment	Fee-for-service	Value based (outcomes, utilization, total cost)
Financial incentives	Do more, make more	Perform better on measures, make more
Financial performance	Margin per service, procedure (bed, physician, etc)	Margin per life

From Grube ME, Kaufman K, Pizzo JJ. Driving the Transition to Value-Based Care. The Kaufman Hall Point of View. Available at: http://www.hfma.org/brg/pdf/Kaufman%20Hall%20Point%20 of%20View_%20Driving%20the%20Transition%20to%20Value-based%20Care_Final.pdf. Accessed December 2013; with permission. Copyright Kaufman, Hall & Associates, LLC.

THE NURSE NAVIGATOR

The cross-continuum nurse navigator role was developed specifically at CMC for HF, with a goal to direct the course of patient care as they transition from acute to ambulatory care after a HF admission. The nurse navigator is the patient advocate and provides care in a highly supportive and personal manner and also serves as a liaison to ensure that patients and families receive resources and services when needed as a link between inpatient and outpatient care. The role has expanded over the past 3 years to meet various needs of the patient and family at various times over the course of transition. The navigator is responsible for identifying patients who are admitted with HF and visits them while in the acute care setting. Once identified, patients and family members are informed of the purpose and goals of the transition clinic (**Fig. 1**).

HEART SUCCESS TRANSITION CLINIC

The HSTC was developed using a transitional care model to support the cross-continuum care of the HF patient. The nurse navigator enrolls each patient in the program with the first appointment scheduled within 3 to 5 days after discharge and the providers involved (attending, primary care physician, cardiologist) are notified of scheduled follow-up. The patient and family meet weekly for 4 to 5 weeks with a HF specialty trained multidisciplinary team including an advanced clinical practitioner, certified heart failure nurse, social worker, pharmacist, and dietitian. The care provided over the course of the program includes specialized HF monitoring and assessments, patient education, pharmacy support and education, social work monitoring, management and assistance, diet education and resources. The interdisciplinary resource team of HF specialists monitors, manages, assists, and cares for the patients to avoid readmission for a minimum of 4 weeks after discharge. Some patient interventions developed by the team include a growing, social network of patients that meet monthly at a HF support group facilitated by the social workers and highlighting a wide range of topics relevant to patient care. Before hospital discharge, through a system-wide education grant, the navigators provide digital scales to patients who do not having functioning scales at home to allow for compliance with daily weighings. Patients are then instructed to bring in their daily weight log to each appointment. Patients are also provided with pillboxes and medication bags at their first appointment. The pharmacists meet individually with patients and enhance compliance using various tools for medication management, including proper return demonstration of pill management and organization. After completing the transition program, the patient's care returns to the primary care team and/or general cardiologist (**Fig. 2**).

    The HSTC team ensures the patient's HF condition remains stable as it relates to fluid management and clinical indicators. Evidenced-based protocols and pathways, developed by the HF specialists, guide all patient care. The 4-week time period allows development of proper care plans and education to allow further compliance and understanding from the patient and family, resulting in enhanced self-care management and improved outcomes. The advanced clinical practitioner communicates with the patient's primary care provider throughout the program and at completion, to ensure coordination and comanagement of the patient.

    With executive support and a goal of decreasing readmissions, a second HSTC was implemented at CHS Northeast, a tertiary center 35 miles from the main facility in May 2012. The same staffing plan was implemented and staff were recruited and trained at CMC to ensure standardization of care. This facility has a large population of HF and index admissions of more than 800 a year. Because there is no advanced HF clinic on

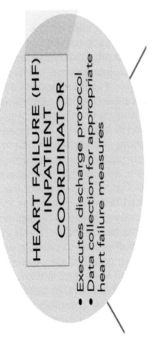
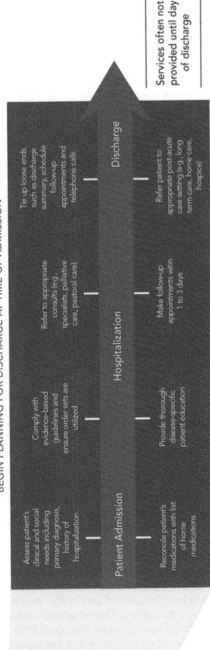

HEART FAILURE (HF) INPATIENT COORDINATOR

- Executes discharge protocol
- Data collection for appropriate heart failure measures

BEGIN PLANNING FOR DISCHARGE AT TIME OF ADMISSION

Patient Admission

Assess patient's clinical and social needs including primary diagnosis, history of hospitalization

Reconcile patient's medications with list of home medications

Hospitalization

Comply with evidence-based guidelines and ensure order sets are utilized

Provide thorough disease-specific patient education

Refer to appropriate consults (eg, specialists, palliative care, pastoral care)

Make follow-up appointments within 1 to 3 days

Discharge

Tie up loose ends, such as discharge summary, schedule follow-up appointments and telephone calls

Refer patient to appropriate post-acute care setting (eg, long term care, home care, hospice)

Services often not provided until day of discharge

Fig. 1. Heart success model: inpatient coordinator. (*Data from* Brown C, Cantril C, McMullen L, et al. Oncology nurse navigator role delineation study. Clin J Oncol Nurs 2012;16:581–5.)

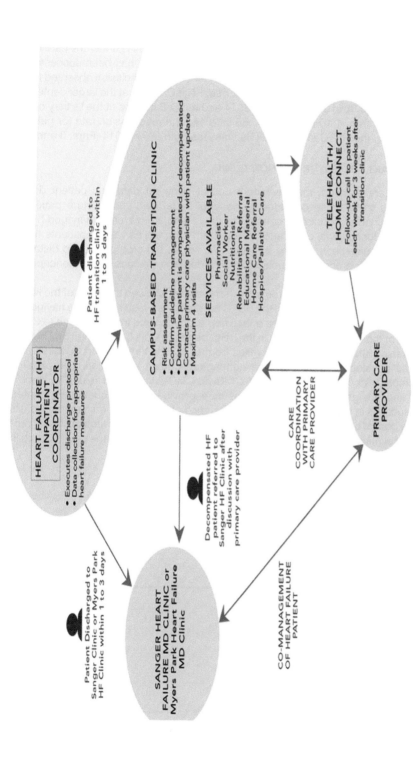

Fig. 2. Heart success model. (*Data from* Brown C, Cantril C, McMullen L, et al. Oncology nurse navigator role delineation study. Clin J Oncol Nurs 2012;16:581–5.)

location, the decision was made to train all nurses in the navigator role. The navigators then rotate between inpatient and the outpatient HSTC, which has provided excellent patient satisfaction with continuity of care because the patient is under the care of the same navigator for majority of the program. Each program has been successful in decreasing readmissions and the global 30-day all-cause readmission observed to expected ratio (O/E) trending down in both facilities. The O/E ratio at the larger center has decreased from 0.98 in 2010 to 0.76 in 2014 and the O/E change at the tertiary center has decreased from 1.10 in 2010 to 0.88 in 2014. The readmission rate for patients participating in the HSTC in both HSTCs was less than 8% in 2014 (**Figs. 3 and 4**).

VIRTUAL HEART SUCCESS TRANSITION CLINIC

As patients are enrolled, the navigators collect pertinent data and patient demographics and track those considered "nonapplicable" and "noncapture patients." The "nonapplicable" population consists of those who are currently managed by the advanced HF longitudinal clinic and/or transplant program as well as patients under the care of hospice services. The patients who refuse the program due to distance, transportation, or comorbidity management interference are considered "noncapture" patients.

In 2012, data from CMC, a quaternary referral center, showed that 30% of the HF index admissions had not enrolled in the HSTC program. As a result, the nurse navigators identified the majority of noncapture due to home location and travel distance to CMC, with many of those patients resided in the neighboring Lincoln County (**Fig. 5**). Through a partnership with CMC-Lincoln (55 miles from CMC) the Virtual Heart Success program was developed to address the noncapture patient population. The patients served receive acute care services at CMC or CMC-Lincoln and reside in Lincoln County and are given the same level of care provided at the quaternary center. CMC's success in improving patient understanding of HF and self-management skills drove the goal of the virtual clinic, to allow patients access to best practice clinical protocols and eliminate travel to tertiary/quaternary center, addressing the potential gap in

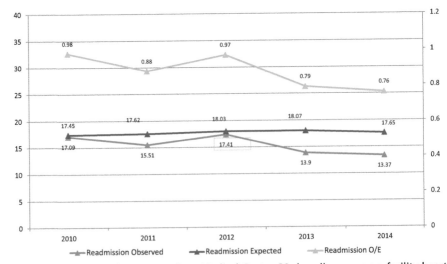

Fig. 3. Carolinas Health Care–Carolinas Medical Center 30-day all-cause same facility heart failure readmission, 2010 to 2014. O/E, observed to expected ratio. (*Courtesy of* Premier, Inc, Charlotte, NC.)

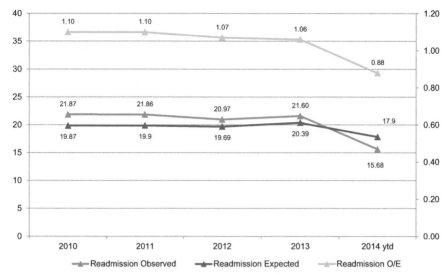

Fig. 4. Carolinas Health Care–Northeast 30-day all-cause same facility HF readmission 2010 to 2014. O/E, observed to expected ratio. (*Courtesy of* Premier, Inc, Charlotte, NC.)

care between the acute care and ambulatory settings. The value creation from this program has shown significant decreases in mileage and hours saved for this patient population as well as an increase in patient follow-up compliance. The volume of patients with a primary diagnosis of HF at the CMC-Lincoln facility did not justify replicating a HSTC in Lincolnton. HF patients discharged from either facility meet with the HSTC team at CMC via telemedicine, using basic videoconferencing and a peripheral stethoscope.[4]

The navigator identifies the patients appropriate for the virtual clinic and collaborates with the inpatient and outpatient case management team to determine patient disposition for transitional care after discharge. The decision was made to allow homebound patients to be seen by home health care workers and to connect virtually with CMC HSTC. Patients not eligible for home health care are scheduled in the SHVI-Lincoln office with a board-certified HF provider. The patient is also connected virtually to the CMC HSTC. In both situations, patients continue with follow-up care within 3 to 5 days of being discharged. The Center for Medicare Services Transitional

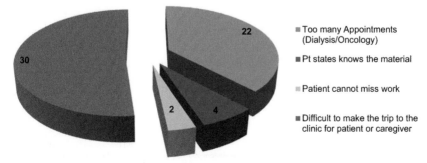

Fig. 5. Heart success: reasons for refusal. Pt, patient. (*Data from* Carolinas Medical Center Heart Failure Nurse Navigator Documentation Tool January through December 2013.)

Care Management E/M code guidelines is being utilized for the virtual patients in the office setting. With the assistance of a home health nurse, the patient is connected to the CMC HSTC's multidisciplinary team via laptop technology from the patient's home or from the SHVI-Lincolnton office. Patients continue to follow-up for 4 weeks after discharge. Provider visit notes are available to the primary care physician and primary cardiologist via the electronic medical record or alternate method if an electronic medical record is not available. Patients are discharged from the transition clinic back to the care of the primary care physician and primary cardiologist at the end of the 4-week transition clinic and may be seen by the primary care physician at any time during the 4 weeks. The home health nurses visit the patient within 48 hours to assess the home situation, start HF education, and apply home monitoring, and are trained to follow the same evidence-based protocols for HF. They identify patients who are high risk for rehospitalization on admission to the home health agency and are trained at the CMC HF clinic to ensure proper patient assessment and documentation.

Although telemedicine is not a new concept, applying it to access specialized advanced care and eliminating travel is innovative and cost effective. As a result of the partnership and collaboration within the system to create the virtual HSTC, patient self-management skills and outcomes have improved. The enthusiasm and excitement of the partnership is evident among all involved through the planning and implementation with a constant goal to improve the outcomes for the HF patients in Lincoln County and proven by a dramatic decrease in readmissions at CHS-Lincoln within 1 year of implementation (**Fig. 6**).

STANDARDIZATION OF PATIENT EDUCATION

Overall, the 3 HSTCs have been successful programs in 3 CHS facilities of different sizes and locations: Carolinas Medical Center (CMC quaternary), CHS-Northeast (tertiary), and CHS-Lincoln (regional). Each facility has a noncapture population that does not participate in the Heart Success Transition programs and the readmission rates are higher in that particular subset of patients. The goal within the past year was to further focus on decreasing readmissions in that population and the navigators

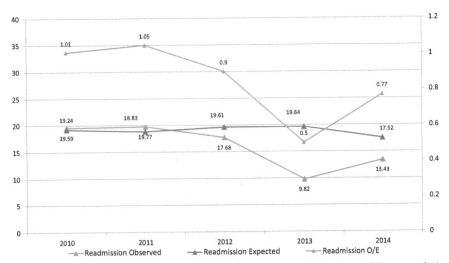

Fig. 6. Carolinas Health Care–Lincoln 30-day all-cause same-facility heart failure readmission, 2010 to 2014. O/E, observed to expected ratio. (*Courtesy of* Premier, Inc, Charlotte, NC.)

worked together with the inpatient staff to enhance and standardize patient education before discharge. The navigators found that the education of HF patients was handled differently in each facility. Patients were being given education material that did not meet national health literacy guidelines and the information differed across facilities. When health literacy is compromised, patient understanding and safety are compromised, resulting in poor health outcomes.[5] If the patient does not understand the necessary self-management tools, including signs and symptoms of HF and when to call the provider (5-year survival for HF patients is 50%), success is not probable and there is a greater risk for readmission. As a result, the navigators from the quaternary and tertiary centers collaborated to design the "What Is Heart Failure" group visit. The group visit model[6] was implemented in the acute care setting to reach the non-capture population before discharge. Patients who meet criteria for attendance include any patient admitted with a primary or history of HF. The navigators identify patients and the appropriate staff is notified to ensure arrival time. Planning and implementation teams, chaired by the navigator, consisted of physicians, clinicians, and administrators from both acute and ambulatory care teams from CHS-CMC and CHS-NE. Both facilities provided staff and time to address the needs of patients with HF to decrease the need for rehospitalization. After receiving approval from the system patient education committee for meeting patient literacy guidelines and appropriate evidence-based criteria, the navigators engaged further disciplines that could assist in patient understanding, including the inpatient diet technician, cardiac rehabilitation, and sleep services for appropriate sleep apnea education. Education of these patients is a priority to improve patient self-management and understanding of their chronic illness.

GROUP VISIT MODEL IMPLEMENTATION

The group visit model was chosen after the success of implementing the group visit model in the HF clinic at CHS-CMC. Shared medical appointments (SMA), a type of group visit for HF had been in place for 2 years and shown to increase productivity, patient access, and efficiency. The SMA visit in the HF clinic has delivered high levels of patient and provider satisfaction. The patient satisfaction survey has received top box results (86.7%). The group visit is a medical appointment in which the provider in a supportive group setting sees multiple patients simultaneously. The advantages of group visits include the ability for patients to assist and teach each other successful coping strategies by sharing personal experiences and providing helpful information. The visit also provides education by the interdisciplinary team as part of the health care experience.

The HF group visit is held 3 days a week and both acute and ambulatory care clinicians share the responsibility of patient attendance and compliance. The HSTC navigators and HF clinic nurses are able to facilitate the class. The nurses teaching the classes are all certified in HF nursing. The group visit addresses all learning techniques with various teaching styles. The visit includes a 15-minute health education video endorsed by the American Association of Heart Failure Nurses entitled, "What Is Heart Failure," and a brief presentation reviewing HF basics.[7] The discussion covers the type of HF, keys to managing HF, medication review, eating with HF, signs and symptoms of HF, and when to call the provider. There is also a presentation on low-sodium diets by the dietetic technician.

It remains the primary nurse's responsibility to provide education to their patients; however, if the patient attends the group visit, the education is provided and documented by the navigator. Class attendance is logged and 30-day readmission is being tracked.

The cross-continuum team has been engaged in the development of the patient education materials to ensure the curriculum is uniform at both facilities. Before implementation of the HF group visit, the classes were held for clinicians in the cardiac service line. This education was an effort to standardize the patient education for HF patients. If a patient or family member is unable to attend one of the group visits, the primary care nurse provides the patient education using the same materials. The primary care nurse is responsible for engaging the patient and family members and inviting them to attend the group visit class. A group visit education brochure, designed by the navigators, is completed by the inpatient nurse or navigator before the visit and includes HF education, including the patient's current HF medicine/s. This documentation allows the facilitator of the class to answer specific questions regarding medications. The education is documented in the patient's record during the class.

The patient feedback has been extremely positive as they learn, challenge, and support one another. Because the HSTC follows patients with a primary diagnosis of HF, the visits allow the clinicians to also reach patients with a secondary diagnosis or history of HF. The group visits have eliminated duplication of efforts and standardization of the materials being used. The educators reach a group of patients at the same time instead of visiting each patient individually, which increases the number of patients reached in less time, and therefore allows the clinician to interact with more patients. With the introduction of cardiac rehabilitation during the class, more patients are engaging in the cardiac rehabilitation program. The group visit model for classes is early in its implementation, but the readmission for this population is trending down. All-cause readmission for the patients that attended the group visit was less than 5% at both facilities. The data are limited, but the team is hopeful for continued improvement in this area. The visit is now a prerequisite for the HSTC, which allows the clinic nurse to apply appropriate "teach back" questions to assess patient's understanding of the material presented. The teach-back process is a successful, evidence-based strategy used to empower nurses to verify understanding, correct inaccurate information, and reinforce teaching with patients and families.[5] The team has discovered that the best way to engage patients in the visit is to provide information that will address their questions, struggles, and fears. Flexibility within the class from the facilitator allows time to address questions, which is an important component of creating a personal, meaningful experience for the patients.

The HF education initiative was completed with no increase in full-time equivalent or staff hours. The group visit model also increases staff efficiency in managing already busy schedules by meeting the complex needs of the chronically ill HF patients with mind and body interventions. The visit is a support group in addition to offering education and allows the cardiac rehabilitation nurse, the primary care nurse, the nurse navigators, and the dietitian to reach multiple patients at the same time, which has strengthened relationship and collaboration between the disciplines. The initiative eliminated duplication of efforts to develop the educational materials and at the same time standardized the tools across facilities. Most important, the initiative addressed the needs of the patient without interruption in the continuum of care. The acute care and ambulatory care teams become "one."

Group visits and SMA offer a creative approach to effective management of high-risk, high-cost patients with chronic conditions. It is proving especially effective in population management of HF patients. The HF SMA is now being offered to pulmonary hypertension patients in the HF Clinic. Plans are to expand the SMA to patients with ventricular assist devices and hospital follow-up visits with patients being managed by the longitudinal HF clinic in 2015. By seeing these patients in a group setting and not using the clinic examination rooms, access for new patient referrals improves. Capacity and demand do match in many practices, and this alternative offers a way to meet increasing needs without adding provider, staff, and space resources. All of this is attained through improved efficiency in managing these complex patients.

The HF team has been partnering with internal and external system programs to share the advanced HF therapy and transitional care outcomes. The teams visited have also been invited to CHS-CMC for site visits to learn more about management of HF. The guests visit the clinic and observe a virtual heart success visit, an SMA, and now the group visit class. The HF nurse navigators are currently partnering with the advanced illness management (AIM) team, a dietitian from the diabetic team, the CMC dietetic technician, and the dietitian from the CHS-NE Heart Success Clinic to evaluate, develop, and standardize teaching tools for nutrition to include recipes and shopping lists for patients.

The group visits model has proven to be an excellent management tool and is assisting HF patients to better self-manage their care. Progress on the initiative and outcomes has been shared with the cardiac service line at both facilities. The lessons learned at CHS-CMC and CHS-NE has enabled the teams to develop a plan to deliver the same care across CHS. Plans for implementation at CHS-Lincoln have started. The CHS-Lincoln patient noncapture percentage has increased and the readmission O/E has increased. The readmission rate is well below the national average, but the CHS-Lincoln navigator has attended and observed the group visit at CMC and has all the same materials to offer the same group visit model. If the program continues to show decreases in the readmission rate, the initiative is easily shared across CHS facilities.

With advances and growth in the advanced HF program, the navigator role has evolved with the demands of the patients. Although data have shown consistently the effectiveness of the role and the program on compliance and decreases in readmissions, the true value of the role is evident by the relationships and trust established with each patient seen. The chronic illness of HF can deprive patients of their overall quality of life. Using a pretest and posttest design, the patient takes a survey on the first and final visit to assess the impact of the program on their quality of life. Results found a decrease in the physical and emotional effects of HF and quality of life. The nurse navigator establishes a relationship of trust and reliance for patients to feel secure and ensured of constant support when needed over the course of their transition. Patients find great satisfaction and security in the nurse navigator, knowing they have a resource to call with questions, concerns, or necessary interventions. The role has proven to be a necessary and warranted position within the HF population and will continue to evolve with the various changes associated with transitional care management. Future plans for expansion of the role include navigator use for acute myocardial infarction and coronary artery bypass graft patients at high risk for readmission and 90-day mortality.

The job summary and responsibilities have expanded with this evolution. The current job description is found elsewhere in this article.

HEART FAILURE NURSE NAVIGATOR
Job Description

Position summary
The Heart Success Nurse Navigator plays a key role in coordination of patients care and therefore increases the efficiency and quality of care that is, delivered. The navigator will provide patient education, support, and direction in a complex multidisciplinary setting.

The navigator will utilize experience, knowledge and skill to facilitate care for patients with HF.

Patient education

- Provides language specific education, psychosocial support, and necessary resources to the patients and their families. Coordinates appropriate referrals for needed services.
- Provides education at an appropriate health literacy level.
- Uses teach-back methodology to assess understanding of education.
- Involves family and/or primary support person in education.
- Reviews and remains current in the latest information on changes in HF care and educational information available.
- Encourages patients to keep and update their own medication records.
- Presents general information on the clinical trials program and refers potential and interested patients to appropriate research resources.
- Facilitates "What Is Heart Failure" group visits.

Patient liaison/advocate

- Serves as an advocate for HF patients.
- Serves as liaison between HF patients/families, participating providers, and the transition clinic.
- Ensures and coordinates new patient referrals and scheduling of appointments, and identifies potential gaps as well as the coordination of care for patients returning to their communities for follow-up.
- Refers patient/family to appropriate resources/services, based on needs assessment.
- Enhances patient satisfaction, identifies and trend barriers to care, and conducts service recovery as needed.
- Communicates with the primary care physician or primary cardiologist.

Outreach

- Assists the Heart Failure Director and the Director of Heart Success in providing education to hospital staff members regarding the transition clinic/heart success program.
- Assists (as needed) in education at other CHS facilities regarding the Heart Success Program.
- Assists as needed with HF support group.

Assess patient and family needs

- Assesses patient/families needs for referrals to support programs.
- Assesses patients with HF for emotional and social needs as well as barriers to care, such as health insurance and transportation, and refers to the needed resources.

Quality outcome measures

- Monitors quality and outcomes measures as directed by the Heart Success Team.
- Evaluates and reports data collected that improve the standards of care for HF patients.

Professional and staff responsibilities

- Performs role based on education preparation, certification, and needs of the CHS system.
- Performs job specific to scope of practice, which further defines the knowledge, skills, and abilities required for the position.
- Is responsible for orienting all pertinent staff in the continuum of care on the role of the nurse navigator.
- Serves as a resource for patients and families.
- Serves as a resource for pertinent physician and staff committees to impact care of HF patients.

REFERENCES

1. Navigator. 2015. Available at: http://www.merriam-webster.com/dictionary/navigator. Accessed July 9, 2015.
2. Brown C, Cantril C, McMullen L, et al. Oncology nurse navigator role delineation study. Clin J Oncol Nurs 2012;16:581–5.
3. Alspach J. Slowing the revolving door of hospitalization for acute heart failure. Crit Care Nurse 2014;1:8.
4. Jones A, Hedges-Chou J, Bates J, et al. Home telehealth for chronic disease management: selected findings of a narrative synthesis. Telemed J E Health 2014;4:346.
5. Kornburger C, Gibson C, Sadowski S, et al. Using "teach-back" to promote a safe transition from hospital to home: an evidence-based approach to improving the discharge process. J Pediatr Nurs 2013;28:282–91.
6. Jones K, Kaewluang N, Lekhak N. Group visits for chronic illness management: implementation challenges and recommendations. Nurs Econ 2014;32:118–47.
7. What is heart failure [video]. Hunt Valley (MD): Milner-Fenwick, Inc; 2014.

Ventricular Assist Device and Destination Therapy Candidates from Preoperative Selection Through End of Hospitalization

Diane Doty, MS, BSN, RN, CCRN, CCNS

KEYWORDS

- Mechanical circulation support options • Flow physiology
- Preoperative/patient selection • Intraoperative • Postoperative
- Patient/caregiver education

KEY POINTS

- Mechanical circulatory support (MCS) is 1 therapeutic option to improve end-organ function, survival, and quality of life in patients with heart failure.
- Critical phases of MCS include patient selection, preoperative preparation, intraoperative care, optimize postoperative care, and posthospital education.
- Key aspects of MCS management are hemodynamics, right ventricular function, infection prevention, nutrition, bleeding and device management, using a multidisciplinary approach, and excellent patient/caregiver education.

Heart failure affects roughly 6 million Americans over the age of 20 years to the tune of $30.7 million in medical costs. This volume is projected to increase 46% by 2030 resulting in 8 million people affected by heart failure. By 2030, the cost is predicted to increase by 127% to $69.7 billion.[1] Currently, there are multiple medical treatments for heart failure such as β-blockers, angiotensin-converting enzyme inhibitor therapy, diuretics, spironolactone, and digitalis. In addition, there are procedural and surgical treatments that include biventricular pacemakers and heart transplantation. Even with these advances in treatment, the 5-year mortality rate for heart failure is 50%.[1] Mechanical circulatory support (MSC) offers another therapeutic option to improve a heart failure patient's end-organ function, survival, and quality of life. These devices have significantly matured in recent years thanks to the development of smaller, high-speed, and rotary pumps. There are 3 areas mechanical circulatory support devices are used: bridge to decision, bridge to transplant (BTT), and destination therapy (DT).

Disclosure Statement: The author has no conflict of interest to declare.
Community Health Network, 8075 North Shadeland Avenue, Indianapolis, IN 46250, USA
E-mail address: ddoty@ecommunity.com

Crit Care Nurs Clin N Am 27 (2015) 551–564
http://dx.doi.org/10.1016/j.cnc.2015.07.006
0899-5885/15/$ – see front matter © 2015 Elsevier Inc. All rights reserved.

In bridge to decision, a ventricular assist device (VAD) is used in a patient temporarily until a more definitive therapeutic treatment decision is made or there is a thorough cardiac recovery. Indications for short-term VAD support are severe myocardial infarction, postcardiotomy or decompensated chronic heart failure, and progress to cardiogenic shock. There is a 50% to 70% mortality for this population.[2] Survival depends on the prompt return of adequate systemic perfusion. The immediate goal of therapy is to decrease the ventricular workload, restore cardiac output, and avoid organ failure. The use of a VAD for bridge to decision allows for a stabilization of hemodynamics and systematic perfusion. The VAD support provides time to optimize the patient's condition and develop a plan for therapy.[3]

BTT is the second arena where MCSs are used. There are roughly 4000 people awaiting heart transplantation in the United States. Transplants have an 80% survival rate with 9.1-year average length of survival.[4] A typical transplant candidate waits 4 months for transplantation. Patients who meet transplant criteria or will be a transplant candidate in the future may be implanted with a VAD while awaiting transplantation. According to the International Society for Heart and Lung Transplant 2012 statistics, 40% of heart transplant patients were BTT.[5] The physiologic benefit of the VAD in these patients are 2-fold. First, there is a decrease in preload resulting in a decrease in the heart's workload. In addition, there is a decrease in the need for myocardial oxygen consumption. Second, the pump maintains a consistent and adequate cardiac output, resulting in systemic circulation augmentation. All of this support gives a damaged myocardium an opportunity to recover. Cardiac assist devices for BTT support patients who are in a premorbid state of organ failure and may successfully return these high-risk patients to a more stable state.

DT is the third venue for MCS. Since the approval of continuous flow HeartMate II for DT, there has been a 10-fold increase in left VAD (LVAD) implants for lifelong support in patients not eligible for a heart transplant.[6] The INTERMACS registry confirmed the superior survival of continuous flow LVADs at 83% at the 1-year mark.[7] The advancement of design and positive clinical trials has led to devices capable of long-term and permanent circulatory support.[6] Long-term heart failure patients experience repetitive heart muscle damage that over time can no longer be treated medically or surgically. The LVAD is designed for this patient population. It provides increase cardiac output; improves cardiac index, hemodynamics, renal and hepatic function, right ventricular (RV) ejection fraction; decreases peripheral vascular resistant; and normalizes fluid volume load.

PULSATILE/CONTINUOUS FLOW PHYSIOLOGY

There are 2 functional categories for VAD—pulsatile and nonpulsatile. The earlier VADs were pulsatile pumps (**Fig. 1**). It was designed to mimic the native heart. Pulsatile devices contain a blood sac. This sac is filled with blood delivered from the left ventricle and then empties into the aorta. This process produces a palpable pulse and blood pressure. The pumps cycle is unrelated to the native hearts electrical activity. Therefore, if the patient experiences dysrhythmias such as ventricular tachycardia or asystole, there is still a palpable pulse. During times of ectopy, the pump fills more slowly related to reduced delivery of blood from the right side of the heart. Pulsatile pumps are preload dependent. The pump's ejection rate depends on the speed at which the blood sac can fill.[8] Pulsatile pumps are used today exclusively in the role of BTT where biventricular support is required. These devises provide an easier transition from an LVAD to biventricular support should RV failure develop.[6]

Continuous flow pumps are the second type of VAD. Continuous flow devices transmit flow through both the systolic and diastolic phases of the cardiac cycle[8] (**Fig. 2**).

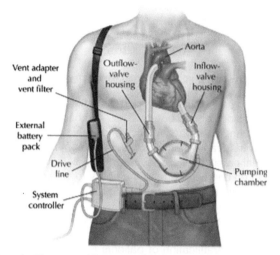

Fig. 1. HeartMate pulsatile pump. (*Courtesy of* Thoratec Corporation, Pleasanton, CA; with permission.)

These pumps are placed with the inlet in the left ventricle and the outlet in the ascending aorta. Most of the blood flows into the pump during systole when the left ventricle ejects into the pump. The pressure difference between the ventricle and the aorta is small. Therefore, patients have lower systolic and greater diastolic

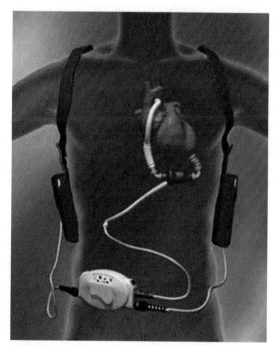

Fig. 2. HeartMate II continuous flow pump. (*Courtesy of* Thoratec Corporation, Pleasanton, CA; with permission.)

pressures resulting in diminished pulse pressures. The usual pulse pressure width for these patients is around 5 to 15 mm Hg.[8] These nonpulsatile devices have changed the face of heart failure treatment and gained support for DT because of their significant survival rate, performance, and smaller size.

PATIENT SELECTION AND PREOPERATIVE CONSIDERATIONS

The selection of candidates for LVAD support is a critical and key to successful implantation. Careful consideration to potential risk and benefits must be taken into account when deciding candidates' acceptance and timing of device implant. There are a multitude of issues that can impact successful outcomes of a patient after device implantation. Potential candidates are assessed on 3 categories: appropriateness of LVAD support based on degree of illness, the ability to undergo the operative procedure successfully, and the ability to be discharged home with adequate family/caregiver support for long-term success.

The Randomized Evaluation of Mechanical Assistance in Treatment of Chronic Heart Failure (REMATCH) trial using the Seattle Heart Failure Score concluded that there is a benefit to risk stratification of patients into low, medium, or high risk for LVAD support.[9,10] This study indicated increase in New York Heart Association class, ischemic etiology, white blood cell count, creatinine, uric acid, cholesterol, and decreased ejection fraction, systolic blood pressure, sodium, hemoglobin, and lymphocyte percentage each had an independent mortality predictive capability[10] **(Table 1)**.

The Interagency Registry for Mechanically Assisted Circulatory Support (INTERMACS) registry, which follows long-term MCS patients in the United States, has identified profiles that help to identify risks associated with the timing of implant. Cardiogenic shock has been identified to have the lowest survival data for patients who receive pulsatile devices. This life-threatening medical condition is the result of ventricular failure most likely related to myocardial infarction. Depending on the severity of the infarction, a patient's ventricles may be unrecoverable, their hemodynamics and vital organ function may be unstable, and there may be irreversible organ damage. In the post REMATCH study it was identified that severe deterioration in general medical condition, poor nutritional status, low serum albumin level, impaired renal function, and right heart failure markers such as low pulmonary artery pressures or increased liver enzymes were at a high risk of in-hospital mortality after LVAD implantation.[11] The INTERMACS data supports the practice of implantation of LVAD early in the progression of heart failure when the patient is more stable.[7] Inotropes may be used to assist with patient stabilization. Inotropes increase intracellular calcium concentrations, which results in increased cardiac output for the heart failure patient.

Table 1 Indicators for increased risk of patient mortality	
Increased	**Decreased**
New York Heart Association class	Ejection fraction
Ischemic etiology	Body mass
White blood cell count	Systolic blood pressure
Creatinine	Serum sodium
Uric acid	Hemoglobin
—	Lymphocytes

The inotropes most commonly used are dobutamine and milrinone. Dobutamine is a β-adrenergic agonist that increases intracellular calcium and myocardial contractility. Milrinone inhibits phosphodiesterase type III, resulting in increased cyclic adenosine monophosphate production, and increases intracellular calcium resulting, in increased contractility. Patients who are stable on inotropes have the best survival.[7]

Nutrition

Malnutrition is seen commonly in patients with congestive heart failure. Roughly 50% of heart failure patients experience weight loss.[12] Patients with weight loss have an increased risk of reduced immune function, skeletal muscle atrophy, prolonged hospitalization, and increased morbidity and mortality.[12] Patients who require MCS are at an increased risk of poor nutrition before implantation. Typically, these patients are admitted to the hospital with worsening heart failure symptoms such as cardiac cachexia. Cardiac cachexia is characterized by the loss of fat and muscle mass and is a profound state of malnutrition.[13] Markers of severe malnutrition are listed in **Table 2**.

There are several advantages of preoperative nutrition for patients who are severely malnourished. These are maintaining weight, visceral protein, sustained prealbumin levels, and decrease in physiologic stress, which could result in tissue damage.[14] Holdy and colleagues[12] stated that, "a comprehensive preoperative evaluation of the LVAD patient should include a nutrition assessment and formalized plan to initiate and advance nutrition support while addressing the metabolic imbalances associated with heart failure." Finally, the International Society for Heart and Lung Transplant Guidelines for Mechanical Circulatory Support: Executive Summary[15] recommends "all patients should have assessment of their nutritional status prior to MCSD implementation with at least a measurement of albumin and prealbumin."

Hemodynamics

Heart failure patient's comorbidities generally are the result of acute or chronic low perfusion and/or congestion. Optimizing a patient's hemodynamics preoperatively may improve the patient's postoperative condition and survival. Increasing cardiac output and cardiac index with the use of inotropes, diuretics, and/or intraaortic balloon pump support improves all organ systems conditions.[16] Slaughter and colleagues[16] identified key strategies such as reducing the central venous pressure (CVP) to 15 mm Hg or less, increasing cardiac index with vasodilators, inotropes, and use of an intraaortic balloon pump in addition to decrease pulmonary vascular resistance with medication such as angiotensin-converting enzyme inhibitors, nitroglycerin, nitroprusside, hydralazine, and inotropes.

Table 2 Severe malnutrition indicators	
Indicator	**Cutpoint**
Body mass index	<20 kg/m^2
Albumin	<3.2 mg/dL
Prealbumin	<15 mg/dL
Total cholesterol	<130 mg/dL
Lymphocyte count	<100
Purified protein derivative skin test anergy	

Infection Prevention

Infection prevention must be a strategic goal for patients who are to undergo LVAD insertion. Chinn and colleagues[17] stated that, "postoperative surgical site infections involving the LVAD develop in 46% of patients, suggesting that the majority of infections occur early on and that the risk of infection increases with the duration of device use." Preoperatively, LVAD candidates may depend on a variety of devices that all have a potential for infection, such as central lines, dialysis catheters, Foley catheters, and ventilators. These devices all can lead to central line blood stream infections, catheter-associated urinary tract infection, and ventilator-associated pneumonia. In addition, patients who are severely hemodynamically unstable are susceptible to developing decubiti, which may become infected. These patients are also vulnerable to several hospital-acquired conditions such as multidrug-resistant microorganisms and *Clostridium difficile*. Strict adherence to evidence-based infection prevention principles such as handwashing, surgical technique, central line, Foley and surgical site care, and prophylactic antibiotic regimen should be a primary goal of all who care for this patient population. Slaughter and colleagues[16] state that, "Limiting device-related infections remains crucial to improving long-term morbidity with survival with implantable LVADs. Adherence to evidence-based infection control and prevention guidelines, meticulous surgical technique, and optimal postoperative surgical site care form the foundation for LVAD associated infection prevention."

Psychosocial Considerations

The ultimate successful outcome for the VAD patient depends on the preparation of the patient and their caregivers. This is life-altering surgery that comes with a unique set of challenges and stressors, such as the fear of managing the device, financial strains, change in family dynamics, and concern with burdening caregivers. The 2013 International Society for Heart and Lung Transplantation Guidelines for Mechanical Circulatory Support: Executive Summary[15] recommends that all MSC patients be screened for psychosocial risk factors, cognitive dysfunction, significant psychiatric illness, and family, social, and emotional support before MCS implantation. VAD patients and their caregivers must have the ability to comply with care instructions, be comfortable with the use and care for the external device, competent to assume responsibility for daily monitoring, device maintenance, and independent performance of activities of daily living.[18]

Exclusion Criteria

The 2013 International Society for Heart and Lung Transplantation Guidelines for Mechanical Circulatory Support: Executive Summary[15] identifies 4 considerations/contradictions for MCS (**Table 3**). Lietz and colleagues[11] stated in the post REMATCH Era implications for patient selection as the following: "Regardless of the type of device, implantations performed in patients with severe functional impairment, end-organ dysfunction and RV failure, malnutrition or infection have been consistently associated with adverse outcomes."

INTRAOPERATIVE CONSIDERATIONS

There are multiple intraoperative considerations for the implantation of a VAD. This article briefly focuses on 4 of those areas.

The first consideration is the management of valvular heart disease. Aortic stenosis that already exists does not significantly affect pump performance. The LVAD decompresses the left ventricle and provides most of the cardiac output. Therefore, this

Table 3 MCS exclusion criteria	
Criteria	**Explanation**
Neuromuscular function	MCS is not recommended for patient's whose neuromuscular disease inhibits their ability to use and care for external device, ambulate, or exercise
Organ failure	MSC is not recommended for patients with irreversible multiorgan failure
Malignancy	MCS is not recommended for patients with active malignancies and a <2-y life expectancy
Pregnancy	MSC is not recommended for patients who are pregnant

From Feldman D, Pamboukian S, Teuteberg J, et al. The 2013 International Society for Heart and Lung Transplantation guidelines for mechanical circulatory support: executive summary. J Heart Lung Transplant 2013;32:161; with permission.

condition does not require correction.[16] Aortic insufficiency does have a significant effect on pump performance for patients who receive a continuous flow VAD. These patients have little to no pulse pressure. The left ventricle contracts, but may not generate enough pressure to open the aortic value. This condition may result in both diastolic and systolic aortic insufficiency, significantly effecting pump performance. Slaughter and colleagues state[16] that "moderate to severe aortic insufficiency warrants a surgical repair or replacement." Mitral valve stenosis also limits the pump's performance, resulting in increased left arterial pressures. Increased left arterial pressures may cause pulmonary hypertension and RV dysfunction. Slaughter and colleagues[16] state that "mitral stenosis needs to be corrected at time of LVAD implant to maximize ventricular filling." Improving right-sided heart function is important in the VAD patient. Because of this, there is consensus that tricuspid insufficiency should be repaired or treated.

The second intraoperative consideration is the proper placement of the percutaneous lead. The placement of this lead is crucial to minimize damage to the lead and, most important, to minimize infection. A discussion with the patient should occur to learn of the patient's hygiene habits and clothing preferences. The percutaneous lead should exit the pump housing with a gentle curve to prevent kinks, which may result in damaged electrical and data cables (**Fig. 3**).

The third intraoperative consideration is the initiation of the pump speeds. Pump speeds are started low at 6000 rpms and increased slowly.[16] The patient must be off cardiopulmonary bypass and there must be complete left ventricle filling before increasing the pump speed. This gradual increase ensures that all air is out of the system. A transesophageal echocardiogram should be done to assess for air in the left ventricle or aorta.[16]

The final intraoperative consideration is RV function. Prevention is the key in RV function. One such intervention was mentioned: evaluation and repair of the tricuspid value. Another is to maintain normal ventilation and oxygenation to prevent acidosis or hypoxia, which may cause pulmonary vasoconstriction.[19] Inhaled nitric oxide is an excellent vasodilator for the pulmonary vascular bed. A randomized, double-blind study by Argenziano and coworkers[20] showed the hemodynamic benefits of inhaled nitric oxide in LVAD recipients with pulmonary hypertension. Inotropes such as milrinone, epinephrine, or vasopressin may be used with moderate RV dysfunction. Finally, maintain a CVP of less than 16 to 18 mm Hg to avoid RV volume overload.[16]

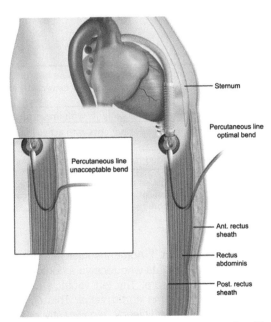

Fig. 3. Percutaneous lead placement. Ant., anterior; Post., posterior. (*Courtesy of* Thoratec Corporation, Pleasanton, CA; with permission.)

POSTOPERATIVE CONSIDERATIONS

Immediate postoperative care for the LVAD patient is not much different from the management of postoperative cardiac surgery patients. There are some particular postoperative consideration for the LVAD patient such as hemodynamics, bleeding and anticoagulation, infection prevention, nutrition, and RV function.

Hemodynamics and the Ventricular Assistance Device Patient

There are 3 key factors to optimize a patient's hemodynamic status: preload, afterload, and contractility. To optimize the VAD pump output, focus must be on improving preload and decreasing blood pressure and afterload (**Table 4**).

All MCS devices depend on preload. Multiple factors can cause a decrease in preload, such as hypovolemia, bleeding, diuresis, vasodilatation, and extravascular fluid shift. A CVP postoperatively should be maintained between 10 and 15 mm Hg for optimal preload.[16] When the fluid balance is negative, pump flow decreases without changes in speed.[21] Initial treatment of low flows is the delivery of intravenous fluids such as colloids, crystalloids, or blood.

Table 4
VAD postoperative hemodynamics

Parameter	Ideal	Complications
Mean arterial pressure	70–80 mm Hg	>90 mm Hg is hypertension
Central venous pressure	10–15 mm Hg	>20 mm Hg consider right ventricular failure
Pulmonary capillary wedge pressure	10–15 mm Hg	—
Mean pulmonary artery pressure	—	>25 mm Hg potential for pulmonary hypertension

Afterload can significantly decrease cardiac output in continuous flow devices and is measured by pulmonary artery and systemic vascular resistance. Increased afterload is the result of increased vascular tone, which can be treated with vasodilators or an obstruction of flow on the outlet side of the pump.[21] There are various causes of outlet obstruction: clot formation, a cannula kink, or tamponade. All of these causes of obstruction require an echocardiogram to confirm diagnosis and requires the patient to return to the operating room for treatment.[21]

Continuous flow devices have minimal pulsatility; therefore, it is difficult to palpate a pulse or measure blood pressure accurately. Early in the LVAD postoperative period, an arterial catheter is necessary to monitor blood pressure accurately. After removal of the arterial catheter, using a Doppler and sphygmomanometer is the most reliable method to assess the patient's blood pressure. Slaughter and colleagues[16] state that, "The goal is maintain the mean arterial blood pressure (MAP) in the range of 70–80 mm Hg." A MAP of 90 mm Hg or greater is defined as hypertension. Vasoactive and inotropic medication and intravascular fluid management can be used to manage arterial blood pressure. The administration of pain medication and sedation may also assist with controlling hypertension in the VAD patient.

Contractility is the third component for ideal cardiac output. Dysrhythmias directly affect the heart's ability to contract. Heart failure patients most likely have preexisting dysrhythmias, such as atrial fibrillation. Patients who undergo any cardiac surgery are also prone to dysrhythmias related to trauma, infarction, electrolyte imbalances, and medication. The VAD patient has an added risk for dysrhythmias related to the risk of ventricular collapse or suction events caused by lack of adequate preload. This causes an increase in negative pressure generated by the pump causing the left ventricle wall to be sucked over and covering the pump's inlet cannula.[21] When this occurs, the ventricular tissue becomes irritated resulting in arrhythmias such as ventricular tachycardia. Dysrhythmia severely compromises the right side of the heart's ability to delivery fluid to the left side. Over time, if preload is not restored the dysrhythmia becomes more sustained and severe. Ways to resolve the issue are to decrease the pump speed and add intravascular volume.[8]

Right Ventricular Function

RV heart failure in LVAD patients is associated with high morbidity and mortality. The ability of the VAD in effectively unloading the left ventricle and increasing preload return to the right side of the heart may overwhelm the right ventricle. A decrease in flow, increase in CVP and pulmonary artery pressures, and deteriorating renal and hepatic function are all indicators of decreasing right side heart function. Some common causes of right sided-heart failure are fluid overload, increased pulmonary vascular resistance, arrhythmias, and ischemia.[22] The goal of treatment for impaired RV function is to reduce afterload and/or increase RV contractility (**Box 1**).

Box 1
Evaluating and managing right ventricular function

Optimum pump speed

  8600 to 9800 rpms for Heartmate II

  Avoid high pump speeds

  Adjust pump speed so aortic valve opens every second or third beat

Echocardiography routinely

Administration of pulmonary vasodilators such as inhaled nitric oxide or intravenous prostacyclin and inotropic medications assist in decreasing afterload. Adequate ventilation must be assessed carefully in VAD patients to maintain normal gas exchange. Such conditions as hypoxemia, hypercarbia, and acidosis may increase pulmonary vascular resistance leading to an increase workload on the right side of the heart.[22] A right VAD may be required if the patient does not respond appropriately to first-line therapy.

Anticoagulation and Bleeding

Anticoagulation therapy is required with continuous flow LVADs to avoid thrombotic complications. Before anticoagulation is started, adequate hemostasis must be achieved and anticoagulation therapy must be modified with changing clinical situations.[16] For example, patients with atrial fibrillation, an artificial heart valve, or low VAD flow rates may need increased anticoagulation therapy.[23] Clinical signs of a potential pump thrombus include tachycardia, dyspnea, increased pulse pressure, and hemolysis. A complete pump occlusion causes a reduced flow rate. Treatment for these issues includes intensive anticoagulant or antiplatelet infusion, local thrombolytic infusion into the device, and reoperation and pump exchange.[8] Postoperative intravenous heparin for anticoagulation may not be needed in all postoperative VAD patients. A 2010 study by Slaughter and colleagues[16] indicated that, "patients who do not receive early postoperative anticoagulation therapy with intravenous heparin as a transition to warfarin and aspirin therapy are not at any early risk for thrombotic events, and their risk of postoperative bleeding is reduced." The literature suggests an International Normalized Ratio of less than 1.5 increases the risk of thrombotic events and recommends adjusting warfarin dose to an International Normalized Ratio range of 1.5–2.5.[24]

Bleeding is a common complication for postoperative VAD implantation and among the most common complications of continuous flow devices. There is an added difficulty in handling bleeding in the VAD population related to their chronic heart failure. By the time a patient receives a VAD implant, their chronic heart failure has affected their kidneys and liver, which can result in altered coagulability after implant. The 2010 study by Slaughter and colleagues[16] stated that, "Patients who receive intravenous heparin in transition to warfarin therapy have the same risk of thrombotic events, but are at an increased risk of post-operative bleeding requiring transfusions." Anticoagulation therapy should be delayed until postoperative bleeding has slowed or stopped.

Gastrointestinal Bleeding

Patients who receive a continuous flow pump are at a greater risk of gastrointestinal bleeding. The flow and the intermittent or absent pulsatile flow cause a narrow pulse pressure and does not allow enough time for clot formation.[25] A study by Crow and colleagues[25] stated that, "the nonpulsatile early and late gastrointestinal bleeding rates where 7 to 10 times higher respectively than were pulsatile bleeding rates." There are multiple causes for gastrointestinal bleeding, such as hemorrhagic gastritis, arteriovenous malformations, driveline erosion, colon polyps, fistulae, and acquired von Willebrand disease. There are several ways to treat gastrointestinal bleeding in the VAD patient. First, discontinue anticoagulation and antiplatelet medications. Second, decrease the LVAD pump speed. These measures increase pulsatile flow and open the aortic value with each beat. The result of these first 2 initiatives is an increase in pulse pressure to allow time for clot formation. Third, initiate a peptic ulcer prevention protocol by starting a proton inhibitor.

Infection Prevention

Infection is among the most common complications in postoperative patients. In the immediate postoperative period, VAD patients have endotracheal tubes, chest tubes, multiple intravenous catheters, intraarterial lines, and catheters. All of these devices put the patient at risk for developing localized or septicemic infections. Significant care must be taken to ensure and maintain asepsis of all invasive lines and catheters. The most critical components of infection prevention must focus on the percutaneous driveline, nutrition, and patient education.[17]

Infection of the percutaneous driveline is a major cause of morbidity and mortality for the VAD patient. Percutaneous drivelines exit from the chest wall or abdomen and are a frequent site for infection for multiple reasons. Trauma at the lead exit site may lead to erythema, which could represent cellulitis. Signs and symptoms of a percutaneous infection are given in **Box 2**.

If an infection at the driveline site is suspected, a culture and Gram stain should be obtained.[17] Immobilization of pump cannulae and leads is key in preventing infection. The International Society of Heart and Lung Transplantation Guidelines for Mechanical Circulation Support Executive Summary[15] recommends that, "The driveline should be stabilized immediately after the device is placed and throughout the duration of support." Immobilization of the driveline may be accomplished with the use of abdominal binders or drain tube holders. The dressing at the percutaneous site should be changed routinely and when saturated. This should be done using sterile technique with the clinician performing the procedure wearing surgical cap, mask, and sterile gloves. The International Society of Heart and Lung Transplantation Guidelines for Mechanical Circulation Support Executive Summary[15] recommends that, "A dressing change protocol should be immediately initiated post-operatively." Finally, the patient and caregiver will be doing the dressing change upon discharge and must receive education and in return demonstrate proper clean technique of dressing change.

Most VAD patients present with severe signs of malnutrition preoperatively. The literature has shown patients who are malnourished have a higher risk of postoperative morbidity and mortality. Nutrition must be addressed as soon as possible postoperatively to ensure adequate protein and caloric intake to promote wound healing.[17] Enteral nutrition is the preferred method of nutritional support of the postoperative VAD patient because it supports gut integrity and can be used to modulate the immune system.[12] Achieving satisfactory nutritional intake is key to maintaining metabolic homeostasis and glycemic control to reduce the risk of infection.

Patient and caregiver education is the third critical component of infection prevention. It is important to educate proper aseptic technique for driveline dressing changes. The patient and caregiver must be educated on the importance of immobilizing the driveline to prevent injury or irritation to the site. Finally, provide education on changes at the driveline exit site that indicate a potential infection and when to notify their health care team.

Box 2
Signs and symptoms of percutaneous drive line infection
Fever
Drainage
Progression of erythema
Leukocytosis

Device Management

Optimization of the patient's VAD pump depends on the parameters of speed, power, pulsatility index, and flow. First, flow and power elements are closely related with the reported flow being an estimate of power and pump speed.[16] There is a direct relationship between flow and power. An increase in power results in an increase in flow. If there is no direct correlation, then there is an issue. Slaughter and colleagues[16] gave multiple examples showing probable thrombus formation. For example, an increase in power that does not result in an increase in flow, an increase in power without an increase in speed, no increase in volume status, no decrease in afterload, and/or a decrease in flow resulting from an occlusion resulting in a decrease of power. In each of these situations, assessment of the pump output should be performed.[16] Second, the pulsatility index measures the pressure difference between the VAD pump and the patient's own cardiac cycle. It provides an indication of volume status, ventricular function, and heart contractility. For instance, a decrease in the pulsatility index without an increase in pump speed may signal a decrease in blood volume.[16] An increase in contractility related to increased volume, inotropes, and/or myocardial recovery increases a patient's pulsatility index.[16] Third, speed is how fast the impeller of the pump spins and is measured in revolutions per minute (rpm). Optimal pump speed is achieved when cardiac index and left ventricular size are within normal limits, there is no left or right shift of the septum and there is some pulsatility with intermittent aortic value opening.[16] The best method to determine pump speed is to perform a ramped speed study using echocardiography and hemodynamic assessment to determine desired cardiac support for the patient.[16] This procedure is usually done in the operating room. Ideal speed range is 8600 to 9800 rpm.[16]

PATIENT AND CAREGIVER EDUCATION

The determination of how successful the VAD implant will ultimately depend on the preparation of the patient and caregiver for their return to home. Discharge to home preparation must start during the preoperative patient selection phase and follow all the way through to discharge. Proper training of both the patient and community will allow for a smooth transition back into the world outside of the hospital. There are a multitude of factors for post discharge education and this article focuses on just some of these.

Rehabilitation in physical, occupational, and nutritional therapy are key to the patient's recovery. It is strongly recommended that patients continue their physical recovery upon discharge. This may require long-term rehabilitation for patients who still show signs of deconditioning upon discharge. Most VAD patients come into the hospital malnourished and showing signs of cachexia and hypoalbuminemia. Therefore, it is important to periodically check on their nutritional status after discharge, which may include a nutrition consultation.

Upon discharge, patients and caregivers are required to perform routine maintenance on the VAD equipment, including looking at connectors, examining vent filters for dirt/debris, and assessing the status of batteries. VAD patients can shower after the surgical site is healed and must ensure that all components of the VAD are protected with waterproof covers.[18] Patients and caregivers must be able to recognize VAD alerts and alarms and know what action to take for each.[16] These patients must also take their vital signs on a daily basis.

Infection prevention is another area of concern after discharge from the hospital. Actions to prevent percutaneous lead infections must be taught to patients and caregivers. Education on how to change the dressing, how to inspect the insertion site, and what the signs and symptoms of an infection are is important. In addition, education on the need and how to immobilize the percutaneous lead is required. Slaughter and colleagues[16] state that, "Established protocols for inpatient and outpatient percutaneous lead care have proven to be effective for pulsatile devices and should be followed."

Upon discharge, VAD patients may resume their normal activities; however, there are some restrictions. Wilson and colleagues[18] identified the following restrictions: avoid extreme temperatures for prolong time periods, avoid power stations/power lines, and be cautious in places that put them at great risk of infection, such as day-cares, sick individuals, and crowded living conditions. In addition, patients should avoid operating of heavy machinery and contact sports.

The final educational piece for VAD patients and their care givers is with regard to the handling of emergencies. Patients and caregivers need to know how to respond and who to contact for device alarms, changes in vital signs, signs of infection, and bleeding. Every patient should have list of emergency contact numbers with them at all times. Finally, patients should be encouraged to contact their VAD coordinator or physician for any change in condition that may be considered serious.

SUMMARY

The quality of life for patients who suffer from advanced heart failure has improved significantly because of the advanced technology of MSC devices. These advances in MSC devices pose new challenges and opportunities that must be handled by a multidisciplinary team working in tandem with the patient and their supporters. The future holds a projected 46% increase in heart failure patients and a continued shortage of suitable donors. The mechanical circulatory support device and its continual evolving technology have opened the door to an option of lifelong support for patients who are not candidates for heart transplantation.

REFERENCES

1. Mozaffarian D, Emelia J, Go A, et al. Heart disease and stroke statistics-2015 update. A report from the American Heart Association. Circulation 2015;131:e1–294.
2. Goldberg R, Spencer F, Gore J. Thirty year trends in the magnitude of management of, and hospital death rates associated with cardiogenic shock in patients with acute myocardial infarction: a population-based perspective. Circulation 2009;119:1211–9.
3. Meyers T. Temporary ventricular assist devices in the intensive care unit as a bridge to decision. AACN Adv Crit Care 2012;23:55–68.
4. Jurt U, Delgado D, Malhotra K, et al. Heart transplant-what to expect. Circulation 2002;106:1750–2.
5. International Registry for Heart and Lung Transplant Registry 2015. J Heart Lung Transplant 2012;10:1052–64.
6. Stewart G, Givertz M. Mechanical circulatory support for advanced heart failure patients and technology in evolution. Circulation 2012;125:1304–15.
7. Kirklin J, Naflel D, Kormos R. Third INTERMACs annual report: the evolution of destination therapy in the United States. J Heart Lung Transplant 2011;30:115–23.
8. O'Shea G. Ventricular assist devices: what intensive care unit nurses need to know about postoperative management. AACN Adv Crit Care 2012;23:69–83.

9. Levy W, Mozaffarian D, Linker D, et al. Can the Seattle heart failure model be used to risk stratify heart failure patients for potential left ventricular assist device therapy? J Heart Lung Transplant 2009;29:1–10.

10. Levy W, Mozaffarian D, Linder D, et al. The Seattle Heart Failure Model: predictive of survival in heart failure. Circulation 2006;113:1424–33.

11. Lietz K, Long J, Kfoury A, et al. Outcomes of left ventricular assist device implantation as destination therapy in the Post-REMATCH era: implications for patient selection. Circulation 2007;116:497–505.

12. Holdy K, Dembitsky W, Eaton L, et al. Nutrition assessment and management of left ventricular assist device patients. J Heart Lung Transplant 2005;24:1690–6.

13. Nellett M, Gregory M, Lefaiver C. Pilot study evaluates nutrition for patients receiving mechanical circulatory support in the intensive care unit. AACN Adv Crit Care 2012;23:258–69.

14. Huckleberry Y. Nutritional support and the surgical patient. Am J Health Syst Pharm 2004;61:671–82.

15. Feldman D, Pamboukian S, Teuteberg J, et al. The 2013 International Society for Heart and Lung Transplantation guidelines for mechanical circulatory support: executive summary. J Heart Lung Transplant 2013;32:157–76.

16. Slaughter M, Pagani F, Rogers J, et al. Clinical management of continuous-flow left ventricular assist devices in advanced heart failure. J Heart Lung Transplant 2010;29:S1–39.

17. Chinn R, Dembitsky W, Eaton L, et al. Multicenter experience: prevention and management of left ventricular assist device infections. ASAIO J 2005;51:461–70.

18. Wilson S, Givertz M, Stewart G, et al. Ventricular assist devices: the challenges of outpatient management. J Am Coll Cardiol 2009;54:1647–59.

19. Krasuski R, Warner J, Wang A, et al. Inhaled nitric oxide selectively dilates pulmonary vasculature in adult patients with pulmonary hypertension, irrespective of etiology. J Am Coll Cardiol 2000;36:2204–11.

20. Argenziano M, Choudhri A, Moazami N, et al. Randomized double-blinded trial of inhaled nitric oxide in LVAD recipients with pulmonary hypertension. Ann Thorac Surg 1998;65:340–5.

21. Christensen D. Physiology of continuous-flow pumps. AACN Adv Crit Care 2012; 23:46–54.

22. Slaughter M, Yoshifumi N, Ranjit J, et al. Post-operative heparin may not be required for transitioning patients with a HeartMate II left ventricular assist system to long term warfarin therapy. J Heart Lung Transplant 2010;29:616–24.

23. Boyle J, Russell D, Teuteberg J, et al. Low thromboembolism and pump thrombosis with the HeartMate II left ventricular assist device: analysis of outpatient anti-coagulation. J Heart Lung Transplant 2009;28:881–7.

24. Kurien S, Hughes K. Anticoagulation and bleeding in patients with ventricular assist devices. AACN Adv Crit Care 2012;23:91–8.

25. Crow S, John R, Boyle A, et al. Gastrointestinal bleeding rates in recipients of nonpulsatile and pulsatile left ventricular assist devices. J Cardiovasc Surg 2009;137:208–15.

Cardiac Transplantation
Considerations for the Intensive Care Unit Nurse

Ashley Moore-Gibbs, MSN, AGPCNP-BC, CHFN*,
Cindy Bither, MSN, ANP-C, ACNP-C, CHFN

KEYWORDS

- Heart transplantation • Advanced heart failure • Immunosuppressive therapy
- Rejection • Endomyocardial biopsy • Denervated heart

KEY POINTS

- Heart transplantation is indicated for patients with advanced heart failure who remain symptomatic despite receiving optimal medical and device therapies.
- A shortage of available organs has increased the need for life support with a bridge to transplant primarily in the form of left ventricular assist devices.
- Postoperative complications of heart transplantation include right heart failure, conduction abnormalities, and infection.
- Transplant rejection continues to be one of the major causes of death and is most frequent during the first month after heart transplant.
- Immunosuppressive maintenance therapy prevents rejection and most commonly consists of triple-drug therapy in the initial postoperative period.

INTRODUCTION

Considerable progress has been made within the field of heart transplantation following the first successful human heart transplant (HT) in 1967.[1] Since that time, more than 100,000 HTs have been performed worldwide.[1] Heart transplantation has become the preferred therapy for select patients with advanced heart failure (HF) who despite receiving optimal medical and device therapies continue to manifest symptoms. Cardiomyopathy is the primary condition leading to HT. Other etiologies contributing to advanced HF requiring HT are listed in **Box 1**.[2]

HT improves survival and quality of life for patients with advanced HF. A limiting factor to this curative treatment is donor availability. The number of HTs performed

Disclosure Statements: The authors have nothing to disclose.
Advanced Heart Failure Program, Medstar Washington Hospital Center, 110 Irving Street, Adv HF Program, Washington, DC 20010, USA
* Corresponding author. 400 East Park Avenue, Charlotte, NC 28203.
E-mail address: amgnp4@gmail.com

Crit Care Nurs Clin N Am 27 (2015) 565–575
http://dx.doi.org/10.1016/j.cnc.2015.07.005
ccnursing.theclinics.com

Box 1
Common underlying conditions requiring heart transplantation

- Cardiomyopathy
- Ischemic cardiomyopathy
- Valvular heart disease
- Repeat heart transplantation
- Congenital heart disease

---

within the United States has plateaued to approximately 2400 annually, with most transplant centers performing 10 to 19 HTs annually.[2] There has been a decrease in death rates for those waiting for HT following an increase in the number of left ventricular assist devices (LVAD) being performed. Patients with an LVAD are at an increased risk for transplantation. **Box 2** highlights potential complications that may increase the risk of an unsuccessful HT.

Approximately 85% to 90% of HT patients live longer than 1 year following their surgery; with the 3-year survival rate being almost 75%.[2] Critical organ shortages require health care providers to perform a rigorous panel of testing and evaluation on patients before deeming them a HT candidate. Major contraindications for HT are related to medical and psychosocial issues. **Box 3** lists contraindications for HT.

PREOPERATIVE PREPARATION

Once a donor is identified for the recipient, a virtual crossmatch is performed to decrease the chance of rejection. The United Network of Organ Sharing (UNOS) is the national regulatory and organ allocation system where transplant centers list patients waiting for HT. UNOS will list donors' antigens and each center will have a list of the recipient's antibodies. Careful attention is paid to compare the two to see if there will be any interaction. Before arriving in the operating room (OR), the HT candidate is examined and laboratory results are evaluated. If there are any issues suggesting signs of infection or significantly abnormal laboratory values, the surgery will be aborted and the next patient on the list will be evaluated for compatibility of the donated organ. Recipients who are on warfarin preoperatively will have anticoagulation reversal with fresh frozen plasma or vitamin K before arriving in the OR. The risk of bleeding and causing hemodynamic compromise in the patient with a re-do sternotomy has led many centers to implement the use of prothrombin complex concentrate (Kcentra) in conjunction with vitamin K, if there is limited time preoperatively to adequately reverse the anticoagulation. They are typed and screened for

---

Box 2
Left ventricular assist device complications increasing the risk of heart transplantation

- Infection
- Higher antibody levels
- Atriovenous malformations
- Stroke
- Re-do sternotomy

Box 3
Patient contraindications for heart transplantation

Absolute Contraindications

Systemic illness with life expectancy less than 2 years despite heart transplantation (HT), including

- Active or recent solid organ or blood malignancy within 5 years
- AIDS with frequent opportunistic infections
- Systemic lupus erythematosus, sarcoid, or amyloidosis with multisystem involvement that is still active
- Irreversible renal or hepatic dysfunction in patients who are being considered only for HT

Fixed pulmonary hypertension

- Pulmonary artery systolic pressure greater than 60 mm Hg
- Mean transpulmonic gradient greater than 15 mm Hg
- Pulmonary vascular resistance greater than 6 Wood units

Relative Contraindications

- Age older than 72 years
- Active infection other than device-related infection in recipients of a left ventricular assist device (LVAD)
- Active peptic ulcer disease
- Severe diabetes mellitus with end-organ damage
- Severe peripheral vascular or cerebrovascular disease
- Morbid obesity (body mass index >35 kg/m^2) in the adult patient
- Cachexia (body mass index <18 kg/m^2) in the adult patient
- Creatinine >2.5 mg/dL or creatinine clearance <25 mL/min
- Bilirubin >2.5 mg/dL, serum transaminases >3 times normal, international normalized ratio >1.5 off warfarin
- Severe pulmonary dysfunction with forced expiratory volume in 1 second 40% normal
- Recent pulmonary infarct (6–8 weeks before HT)
- Resistant or refractory hypertension
- Irreversible neurologic or neuromuscular disorder
- Active mental illness or psychosocial instability
- Drug, tobacco or alcohol use within 6 months
- Heparin-induced thrombocytopenia within 100 days

Adapted from Fischer S, Glas KE. A review of cardiac transplantation. Anesthesiol Clin 2013;31:383–403.

---

leukoreduced packed red blood cells and platelets, to decrease the antibody transference during transfusion, as this can precipitate a rejection.[3] If the patient is cytomegalovirus (CMV) negative, a request is also made for CMV-negative blood transfusion.[3] CMV conversion from negative to positive can be catastrophic for an immune-suppressed patient and can present as gastritis, pneumonitis, or nephritis.

If the HT recipient has an infected LVAD in place, he or she will go to the OR on the appropriate antibiotics and therapy will continue for a prolonged time, as determined by the infectious disease team at each institution.[4] Before leaving the floor for the OR, the patient also will be given mycophenolate mofetil (CellCept) as the start of their immunosuppressant regimen. Some centers will also administer steroids preoperatively.

PERIOPERATIVE PERIOD

The time in the OR for the HT recipient begins before the donor heart arrives. If the patient has had a previous sternotomy and/or an LVAD, there can be multiple adhesions making entry into the chest difficult. This process can lead to excessive bleeding from the tissue surrounding the heart and the surgeon works to cauterize all areas before closing the chest at the end of the surgery. The recipient's native heart is cleared of adhesions and prepared for removal, so that when the new heart arrives, there is minimal additional ischemic time for the donor heart. After the new heart is sutured in and the patient has come off bypass, a high dose of steroids is administered. Another dose of steroids is given on arrival to the intensive care unit (ICU) and a continued, gradual

---

Box 4
Perioperative interventions and considerations for patients receiving heart transplantation

Perioperative period

- Patient receives mycophenolate mofetil to start the immune-blocking process before going to the operating room (OR)
- Steroids administered in the OR
- All blood products are leukodepleted
  - Leukodeplete transfusions preferred due to the antibodies that are present in white blood cells
  - Cytomegalovirus (CMV)-negative blood is administered to CMV-negative patients to prevent conversion and subsequent sequelae
- Patients usually need chronotropic support due to the stunning of the sinoatrial node from the cold ischemic time and/or right ventricular swelling; chronotropic support can be achieved by
  - Temporary epicardial pacing wires (atrial pacing)
  - Intravenous medications (Isuprel or epinephrine)
  - The heart rate should be no less than 90 to 100 beats per minute
  - Medications that work through the vagal nerve (atropine and digoxin) no longer have the same effect due to denervation
- Right ventricular (RV) failure can be an issue
  - Due to poor preservation during the cold ischemic time
  - Patients who have had LVADs with elevated pulmonary pressures usually show reversal in approximately 6 months, which makes them eligible for transplantation
    - This will still be an issue postoperatively and the RV can fail
    - Vitally important to monitor the central venous pressure with readings in the mid-teen range to prevent secondary organ failure
- Even if the left ventricle (LV) is functioning normally, the RV may need support with initiation of milrinone or other agents such as inhaled Flolan, to decrease the pulmonary pressures making it easier for the RV to empty

dose taper occurs during the ensuing hospital course. **Box 4** provides a summary of interventions and considerations when caring for a HT patient perioperatively.

POSTOPERATIVE PERIOD

The denervated heart will usually require chronotropic support postoperatively. An adequate heart rate is maintained with isuprel, epinephrine, or pacing via the epicardial wires placed at the time of surgery. The target heart rate after transplantation is usually 90 to 100 beats per minute.[3] It is important for the ICU clinician to be aware of certain medications that will not have the desired effect on the denervated heart, such as atropine and digoxin.

A common conduction abnormality seen after transplantation is delay in the sinoatrial (SA) node conduction. With the donor heart ischemic time and packing in cold preservation fluid, there can be a tendency for the patient to have a junctional rhythm postoperatively. Weaning of chronotropic agents will be difficult until conduction via the donor SA node returns. Some recipients may require a single lead pacemaker postoperatively if an adequate heart rate is not maintained.[3] Before a permanent pacemaker, agents such and terbutaline and theophylline can be used to attempt to increase the heart rate; however, these medical therapies are associated with adverse effects, including tremors and agitation.

Another potential postoperative issue that can arise is right ventricular (RV) failure. Registry data from the International Society of Heart and Lung Transplant (ISHLT) indicate that approximately 20% of early deaths following transplantation are attributable to RV failure.[1] If pulmonary artery pressures are elevated preoperatively, this may cause hemodynamic impairment immediately after HT. The RV of the newly implanted heart has not previously been contracting against high pulmonary pressures and can fail once transplanted into the recipient if the pulmonary arterial resistance is too high. This is often seen in a patient who has RV pressure elevation secondary to left ventricular (LV) failure. Before the LVAD era, those patients were either turned down for transplantation or referred for a dual heart-lung transplant. LVAD therapy can be beneficial in the reversal of pulmonary pressures after approximately 6 months of offloading the ventricle.[5] Transplant centers will monitor pulmonary pressures while the recipient is on the waiting list to determine the most appropriate timing for transplantation. During the immediate postoperative period, when the LV is no longer being offloaded, there can be a slight rebound in elevation of pulmonary pressures that can challenge the RV of the implanted heart. Frequently, the HT recipient will be treated with inhaled epoprostenol or milrinone in an attempt to lower the pulmonary pressures. As recommended in the guidelines,[3] there are many other agents, such as nitroglycerin, inhaled nitric oxide, and sildenafil, which can also be used. As the patient approaches a euvolemic state and the RV rebounds, these agents can be weaned off and most of them will recover. Close monitoring of the central venous pressure (CVP) is important to assess for preload and the patient's filling pressures. Low CVP readings should be avoided to prevent end-organ involvement and possible damage. This can be seen with worsening glomerular filtration rate due to a drop in renal perfusion pressure. Serum lactate levels also may be trended to monitor end-organ function. With the addition of calcineurin inhibitors to the medication regimen, renal function may further deteriorate and creatinine trends should be closely monitored. If organ function shows signs of compromise and medical therapy is not altering the clinical picture favorably, a patient likely may be placed on surgical support, such as RV assist device, LVAD, or extracorporeal membrane oxygenation (ECMO), until the organ recovers.[3] Careful timing of these therapies is critical or end-organ recovery may not be possible.

Early extubation and discontinuation of indwelling vascular access and chest tubes is desirable to prevent infection. If prolonged central access is required, it is best to have it placed on the left side, so that the right internal jugular will be spared for future endomyocardial biopsies. Incisional care is transplant center specific, but it is generally recommended to leave dry incisions open to the air to help aide in healing and prevent moisture over the site. Depending on the presence of infection, previous LVAD exit sites are addressed in 1 or 2 ways. If the patient does not have an infected LVAD, the driveline site is closed; however, in the case of an infected driveline, the site will remain open and surgically packed with dressings. The surgeon will usually attempt to remove all of the old driveline remnants in the case of infection but may choose to leave a portion of the noninfected driveline in place. Any extra incisions in the immune-suppressed patient will increase the risk of infection, so transplant center experience will help determine the process undertaken.

Medications in the postoperative period will be initiated as per the transplant center's protocol, but generally steroids will be started preoperatively and perioperatively. Mycophenolate mofetil (MMF) is given preoperatively and then continued postoperatively. Calcineurin inhibitors (CNI) are initiated 24 to 72 hours after the transplant.[3] Induction therapy is received by those transplant recipients who have an antibody mismatch or renal insufficiency. This will allow a longer period of time before starting the CNI, avoiding potential nephrotoxicity. In summary, maintenance therapy most commonly consists of triple-drug therapy, including steroids, a CNI (tacrolimus or cyclosporine), and an antiproliferative agent (MMF or azathioprine). **Table 1** outlines considerations of immunosuppressive therapy for the post-HT patient.

During the first week following HT, the immunosuppressed recipient is also started on agents to provide prophylaxis against relevant common pathogens. A typical regimen will include antifungal agents (nystatin or fluconazole) for thrush prevention, Bactrim (sulfamethoxazole/trimethoprim) for Pneumocystis pneumonia (PCP) prophylaxis, and valganciclovir (Valcyte) to prevent infection with CMV.[3] Of importance to note, the transplant medications should be scheduled carefully to maintain therapeutic levels. The timing of therapeutic drug monitoring by blood sample must be 12 hours following the previous administration to obtain a true trough level. If a patient has nothing-per-mouth instructions, the decision to withhold medications must be thoroughly explored. If there is a prolonged intubation, CNI can be given intravenously (IV) in addition to other IV medications.

Rejection in the ICU typically manifests as hemodynamic instability, the presence of dysrhythmias, or both. Persistent paroxysmal atrial flutter should alert the nurse to notify a provider, as it is a strong marker for rejection.[6] Of note, ventricular arrhythmias have not been linked to rejection.[6] Hemodynamic impairment during a rejection episode will be reflected by worsening LV function, decreased pulmonary artery oxygen saturations, and an increase in filling pressures. An echocardiogram (echo) is immediately obtained when assessing for possible rejection.[6] Depressed LV function on an echo may be evident even before overt clinical manifestations of cardiogenic shock. If suspicion for rejection is confirmed, the patient will undergo endomyocardial biopsy, and high-dose pulse steroids are given as the first-line therapy. The use of inotropic support also may be needed to maintain adequate organ perfusion.

Endomyocardial biopsy assesses for myocardial damage from cellular or antibody-mediated rejection. Diagnosis of cellular rejection is made using the ISHLT grading scale. Biopsies are classified as grade 0 R (no rejection), grade 1 R (mild rejection), grade 2 R (moderate rejection), or grade 3 R (severe rejection).[7] An endomyocardial biopsy returning as grade 2 R or higher is a significant finding, and treatment for rejection is necessary.[7] Antibody-mediated rejection is more difficult to diagnose. The

Table 1
Immunosuppressive therapy in the patient after heart transplantation

Immunosuppressant Class	Mechanism of Action	Side Effects	Therapeutic Range

CNIs
• CSA
• TAC
	Suppresses the activation of T lymphocytes, prevents T-cell–mediated (cellular) rejection	• CSA: HTN, hyperlipidemia, hirsutism, gingival hyperplasia, nephrotoxicity, diabetes mellitus, tremor, GI symptoms, infection
		• TAC: HTN, hyperkalemia, hypophosphatemia, hypomagnesemia, nephrotoxicity, diabetes mellitus, tremor, diarrhea, infection
			Dependent on:
			1. Time from transplantation
			2. Renal function
			3. Other comorbidities
			4. Concurrent immunosuppressive agents
			  • CSA: 12 h trough 100–400 ng/mL
			  • TAC: 12 h trough 5–20 ng/mL

Antiproliferative agents • AZA • MMF • Mycophenolate sodium (Myfortic)	Inhibit T- and B-cell proliferation (cellular and humoral rejection)	• AZA: leukopenia, thrombocytopenia, nausea/vomiting, infection • MMF: nausea, vomiting, diarrhea, leukopenia, infection • Mycophenolate sodium: fewer GI symptoms due to enteric coating, leukopenia, infection	• No therapeutic range for these drugs • AZA: CBC and platelet monitoring due to risk of bone marrow suppression and cytopenias • Mycophenolate: monitor WBCs due to risk of leukopenia

mTOR inhibitors (proliferation signal inhibitors)
• Everolimus
• Sirolimus
	• Inhibit cell proliferation by blocking phase of the cell cycle
	• Inhibit T-cell proliferation
	• Antineoplastic effects
		• HTN, hyperlipidemia, hypertriglyceridemia, thrombocytopenia, anemia, diarrhea, acne, rash, poor wound healing, increased risk of bacterial infections
		• Sirolimus associated with pneumonitis
			Dependent on:
			1. Time from transplantation
			2. Concurrent immunosuppression
			  • Everolimus: 12 h trough 3–8 ng/mL
			  • Sirolimus: 24 h trough 4–12 ng/mL

Corticosteroids • Methylprednisolone • Prednisone	Multifactorial: • Alter RNA and DNA synthesis • Inhibit macrophages and T cells	Hyperglycemia, weight gain, osteoporosis, HTN, hyperlipidemia, cataracts, adrenal insufficiency, fluid retention, muscle weakness, puffiness of face, easy bruising of skin, peptic ulcers, mood disturbances, infection	• None • Dose depends on time from transplantation • May be used for chronic rejection suppression but often in immediate post-transplant period and then for acute rejection

Abbreviations: AZA, azathioprine; CBC, complete blood count; CNI, calcineurin inhibitor; CSA, cyclosporine; GI, gastrointestinal; HTN, hypertension; MMF, mycophenolate mofetil; mTOR, mammalian target of rapamycin; TAC, tacrolimus; WBC, white blood cell.

From Flannery MP, Smith LM. American Association of Heart Failure Nurses: advanced heart failure. Mt Laurel (NJ): AAHFN, in preparation; with permission.

endomyocardial biopsy is assessed for histologic abnormalities, including endothelial activation with macrophages and capillary destruction along with immunologic findings of complement and HLA deposition.[7]

The type of rejection will determine the treatment required. There are 3 types of rejection in the transplanted heart: hyperacute/antibody mediated, cellular, and vascular. Hyperacute rejection primarily occurs very early in the postoperative period, and often while the patient is still in the OR. It stems from antibody-mediated rejection that is brought about by the compliment system. The recipient's antibodies react against the donor heart antigens after implantation. The primary treatments are high-dose steroids, plasmapheresis, and IV immunoglobulin; cytolytic immunosuppressive therapy

---

Box 5
Postoperative interventions and considerations for patients receiving heart transplantation

Postoperative period

- Clinicians will pay close attention to the ischemic time, as the ideal time for graft survival is <4 hours
  - Increased ischemic time will have sequelae of the graft success, as well as patient long-term survival
- A dose of steroids will be administered on arrival to the intensive care unit (ICU)
- The first 24 hours will include careful monitoring of pulmonary artery (PA) pressures and PA saturations to ensure adequate circulation
- Mycophenolate mofetil will be continued in the intravenous (IV) form on a twice-a-day (BID) dosing regimen until the patient is taking oral medications
- Strict isolation is no longer required, but strict hand washing and sterile technique with IV lines and incisions should be stressed
  - Clinical care staff with any sign of infection should not be caring for a transplant patient
  - Any opening, such as an old LVAD driveline exit site, if not closed, should be packed and covered
    - Patients with a driveline infection should have the entire driveline removed and is a question to ask the surgeon during hand off
  - Surgical incision care is center specific
- Early extubation remains the gold standard to prevent hospital-acquired pneumonia
- Calcineurin inhibitors are started on postoperative days 2 to 5; initiation is dependent on whether induction therapy was received
  - Induction therapy is given to the patient who may have an antibody mismatch or the patient with renal insufficiency
    - This will give days of increased immunosuppression with an agent that is not toxic to the kidney
    - Timing of the medication is critical to the efficacy of the medication
  - The primary calcineurin inhibitor at this time is Prograf (tacrolimus)
    - It is initially started in the ICU via IV and converted to oral capsules; recommended that the first dose be given 8 to 10 hours after the IV preparation is discontinued
      - Calcineurin inhibitors are nephrotoxic and creatinine trends must be measured daily until steady-state levels are appropriate for a fresh transplant
      - Calcineurin inhibitors (Prograf) are occasionally used as monotherapy long term, but this is currently seen in only a few transplant centers/patients

- Steroids are converted from methylprednisolone to prednisone and a tapering dose is initiated
    - Each center has specific tapering guidelines, and nurses should be familiar with their own center's protocol
    - It is vitally important that steroids are given on a BID basis, especially early in the postoperative course
    - There is usually an initial rise in white blood cells after steroids are introduced; if the rise seems out of proportion, cultures can be drawn to rule out infection
    - The goal is to totally wean the patient off steroids if there are no episodes of severe rejection (this is usually at or by the sixth postoperative month)
- Due to the level of immunosuppression, the patient is prescribed prophylactic antibiotics, antivirals, and antifungals
- A venous blood test, Immuno, may be ordered to measure the level of immunosuppression that will provide direction if medication dosing adjustments are needed

- Screening for rejection
    - Clinical signs of rejection
        - Atrial arrhythmias
        - Worsening graft function (primarily seen in the LV) and reflected in abnormal LV function and worsening hemodynamics
        - Low-grade temperatures
        - Decreased electrocardiogram voltage
    - Routine screening
        - Endomyocardial (EM) biopsy
            - Looking for cellular rejection and also staining with immunofluorescence for immunologic rejection
            - The first EM biopsy is usually at postoperative week 1
            - It is most often performed via the right internal jugular venous access either under fluoroscopy or echo guidance
            - In the patient who is >3 months out from HT there is a blood test available to monitor the levels of rejection; however, the EM biopsy remains the gold standard for screening
            - Treatment regimen for rejection
                - The first therapy is usually a bolus of steroids (500 mg or 1000 mg depending on the patient body habitus, once daily for 3 days)
                - All drug levels are checked or adjusted to provide increased immunosuppression
                - If all levels and drugs are in the expected range, other therapies can be introduced
                    - Plasmapheresis
                        - Done via a dialysis catheter
                        - The plasma contains increased antibodies that are exchanged during this process with fresh plasma
                    - Rituximab
                        - Instituted at the completion of plasmapheresis, to aid in destroying B cells

agents (antilymphocyte); and the standard immunosuppressive therapy as noted previously.[3] There are times that the recipient will need to be supported with ECMO while therapy is ongoing. Because of the high mortality with this rejection, retransplantation is recommended, but with a minimal success rate.[3] There is also a class of antibody-mediated rejection that is seen farther out from the initial transplant, and that can be found with a biopsy and special staining of endomyocardial tissue.

Cellular rejection is primarily T-cell mediated, as the body mounts a response to the recognition of foreign tissue. T lymphocytes are seen invading the tissue and the extent of the invasion, along with the amount of cardiomyocyte damage, is what the rejection grading system describes. High-dose steroids are again the first-line medication, followed by optimization of target drug levels, and if they are hemodynamically compromised, more aggressive drug therapy will be used. If a HT recipient who is out far enough from transplantation to be off prophylactic medications is admitted with acute cellular rejection, the prophylactic medications will be reinstated.

Cardiac allograft vasculopathy (CAV) varies widely and is not an immediate postoperative complication, but is more commonly seen years following HT. Characteristics of vasculopathy include panvascular disease, generally lipid-poor concentric lesions, arterial constriction, and rapid progression.[7] A large cohort study of more than 2600 patients from 39 institutions demonstrated angiographically significant CAV in 42% of patients at 5 years and 50% at 10 years.[7] CAV can occur as soon as 1 year following HT.[7]

HT recipients do not experience typical angina due to denervation of the transplanted heart, making it difficult to evaluate from a symptom standpoint. Over time, some patients may develop reinnervation of the cardiac muscle and experience chest pain.[7] Routine surveillance with coronary angiography is used to assess for CAV.[7] Prevention is an important strategy, with control of hypertension and hyperlipidemia. Medical therapy often will include antihypertensive medications, HMG-CoA reductase inhibitors (statins), and aspirin. When CAV becomes clinically significant, percutaneous coronary intervention and stenting is performed, although restenosis is common in HT patients.[7] HT patients who are not amenable to percutaneous coronary intervention or coronary artery bypass grafting may be considered for retransplantation.

Box 5 provides a summary of interventions and considerations when caring for an HT patient postoperatively.

SUMMARY

Heart transplantation is indicted for select patients with advanced HF who experience significant symptoms despite optimal maximal drug and device therapies. Advances in immunosuppressive therapy and posttransplant care have significantly improved transplant recipient survival. It is essential for ICU clinicians to have a sophisticated understanding of the management strategies and potential postoperative complications to successfully manage this patient population.

REFERENCES

1. Fischer S, Glas KE. A review of cardiac transplantation. Anesthesiol Clin 2013;31: 383–403.
2. Lund LH, Edwards LB, Kucheryavaya AY, et al. The registry of the International Society for Heart and Lung Transplantation: thirty-first official adult heart transplant report-2014; focus theme: retransplantation. J Heart Lung Transplant 2014;33: 996–1008.

3. Costanzo MR, Dipchand A, Starling R, et al. The International Society of Heart and Lung Transplantation Guidelines for the care of heart transplant recipients. J Heart Lung Transplant 2010;29:914–56.

4. Koval CE, Rakita R, AST Infectious Diseases Community of Practice. Ventricular assist device related infections and solid organ transplantation. Am J Transplant 2013;13:348–54.

5. Mikus E, Stepanenko A, Krabasch T, et al. Reversibility of fixed pulmonary hypertension in left ventricular assist device support recipients. Eur J Cardiothorac Surg 2011;40:971–7.

6. Thajudeen A, Stecker EC, Shehata M, et al. Arrhythmias after heart transplantation: mechanisms and management. J Am Heart Assoc 2012;1:e001461. Available at: http://jaha.ahajournals.org/content/1/2/e001461.short. Accessed May 30, 2015.

7. Kittleson MM, Kobashigawa JA. Management of the ACC/AHA staged patient cardiac transplantation. Cardiol Clin 2014;32:95–112.

Palliative Care in Heart Failure

Judith E. Hupcey, EdD, CRNP[a],*, Lisa Kitko, PhD, RN[b], Windy Alonso, MS, RN[a]

KEYWORDS

- Palliative care • End of life • Heart failure • Family caregivers

KEY POINTS

- Heart failure is a progressive life-limiting disease, with high morbidity and mortality, yet advance care planning, end-of-life conversations, and referrals to palliative care do not occur frequently.
- Palliative care is a philosophy of care focusing on patients and their families from diagnosis through death and bereavement.
- Nurses serve as a bridge to palliative care by providing basic palliative care interventions and recognizing the time for referral to specialized services.
- The 4 overarching components of basic palliative care address issues concerning the patient's emotional, social, spiritual, and physical issues, including uncontrolled symptoms.
- Nurses should be advocates for patients and caregivers by initiating specialized palliative care consults for all patients with advanced heart failure.

HEART FAILURE BACKGROUND

Approximately 5.7 million Americans are diagnosed with heart failure and this number is increasing.[1] It is anticipated that the number of heart failure cases will increase 46% by 2030 to more than 8 million, with the cost surging from $30.9 billion in 2012 to almost $70 billion in 2030. The number of deaths attributed to heart failure also remains high; the numbers virtually unchanged from 15 years ago, with the 5-year mortality rate after initial diagnosis still hovering around 50%. Patients with advanced or stage D heart failure even have a more dismal prognosis.[2] After a hospitalization for an acute exacerbation, there is an 11% chance of death within 30 days of discharge and a 25% chance of readmission within 1 month of discharge.[3]

Although heart failure is a progressive and life-limiting disease with high morbidity and mortality, advance care planning and end-of-life conversations frequently do not

There are no commercial or conflicts of interest for the authors.
[a] The Pennsylvania State University College of Nursing, 1300 ASB/A110, 90 Hope Drive, Hershey, PA 17033, USA; [b] The Pennsylvania State University College of Nursing, Nursing Sciences Building, University Park, PA 16802, USA
* Corresponding author.
E-mail address: jhupcey@psu.edu

Crit Care Nurs Clin N Am 27 (2015) 577–587
http://dx.doi.org/10.1016/j.cnc.2015.07.007
0899-5885/15/$ – see front matter © 2015 Elsevier Inc. All rights reserved.

ccnursing.theclinics.com

occur, as patients, families, and health care providers wait for each other to initiate these discussions.[4–7] One of the recommendations from the landmark (IOM) report, "Dying in America,"[8] is clinician–patient communication with advance care planning (p. S-9), which at present is poor and feeds into the lack of services offered to patients with serious advanced illnesses and lack of advance directives, even with the sickest of patients.[9] These services include both hospice and palliative care, and have been recommended to meet the complex needs of patients and their family caregiver throughout the heart failure trajectory.[10] In addition, when palliative care and hospice are used in the last year of life, the rates of hospitalizations and outpatient visits decreases.[11] The use of these services also is extremely important because heart failure patients are at risk for rapid decline and sudden death.[12,13] However, in-patient palliative care consultations, if done, typically are not being ordered until the last month of life,[14] although the use of these services decreases costs and increases patient satisfaction.[15] Although the percentage of end-stage heart failure patients referred to hospice has significantly increased since 2000, heart disease in general still only accounted for 11.2% of hospice admissions in 2012,[16] with less than 10% of these admissions for heart failure.[13,17] For other medical and therapeutic services (eg, cardiac rehabilitation, occupational therapy, physical therapy) focused on promoting, restoring, and maintaining health, with the goal of maximizing the level of independence, only 4.3% of admissions were for heart failure.[18]

WHAT IS PALLIATIVE CARE?

Palliative care is a philosophy of care and care delivery service that focuses on both patients and their families throughout the trajectory of a life-limiting/serious illness,[10] from diagnosis through death and bereavement. As a philosophy of care, palliative care is delivered across the continuum of health care settings by both certified palliative care specialists and noncertified health care providers.[8] Specialty palliative care is provided by a team of palliative care–certified doctors, nurses, and other specialists who work together with a patient's other doctors to provide an extra layer of support. Basic palliative care is delivered by non–palliative care–certified professionals. These include services provided by primary care providers, subspecialists (eg, cardiologists), nurses, and others health care professionals who care for these patients.

According to The National Consensus Project for Quality Palliative Care the goals of palliative care are:

> to prevent and relieve suffering and to support the best possible quality of life for patients and their families, regardless of the stage of the disease or the need for other therapies. Palliative care is both a philosophy of care and an organized, highly structured system for delivering care. Palliative care expands traditional disease-model medical treatments to include the goals of enhancing quality of life for patient and family, optimizing function, helping with decision making, and providing opportunities for personal growth. As such, it can be delivered concurrently with life-prolonging care or as the main focus of care.[19(p6)]

Specific aspects of palliative care include the prevention and relief of suffering by means of early identification, assessment, and treatment of pain and other problems, whether they be physical, psychosocial, and spiritual.[20] Palliative care is differentiated from hospice in that the focus of palliative care is on patients with a serious illness and can be provided along with life-sustaining treatments. Hospice, which also delivers palliative care, is described as, "a service delivery system that emphasizes symptom management without life-prolonging treatment and is intended to enhance the quality of life for both patients with a limited life expectancy and their families."[21(p2)] The traditional model of palliative care is shown in **Fig. 1**[19]; however, this model shows an abrupt shift from life-prolonging therapy along with palliative care to hospice. Conceptually, this is not accurate because palliative care is an overarching philosophy that includes basic palliative care delivered by all health care providers along with specialty care and hospice as part of the delivery mode of care. **Fig. 2** depicts a more encompassing model of palliative care as both a service model and philosophy of care.

COMPLEXITIES OF HEART FAILURE AND PALLIATIVE CARE

Because heart failure is a life-limiting illness, patients diagnosed with heart failure fit the criteria for the provision of palliative care; however, few patients receive these services.[22] There are many reasons why services are not received, including the unpredictable course of heart failure, which complicates prognostication; failure by health care providers to have advance care planning and end-of-life conversations with patients and families; a lack of understanding of palliative care by providers,[4,23–25] patients, and families[26,27]; and a limited availability of specialized palliative care services.[28,29]

Heart Failure Illness Trajectory: Unpredictable Course

The heart failure illness trajectory is complex and unpredictable.[2,12,30] The unpredictable nature of the illness trajectory is cited as a reason for services not being offered and, if offered, not being accepted by heart failure patients and families. The typical heart failure trajectory is characterized by acute crises followed by periods of stability that may last weeks to months to even years (**Fig. 3**).[31]

The concern with this model is the risk of rapid cardiac decompensation or sudden death. Although there are predictive models available, physicians may not attempt to risk stratify patients, are unfamiliar with these predictive mortality models, or are not comfortable with accuracy of models, and thus do not use them.[17] To complicate risk stratification, predicted mortality can change with advances in medical management, cardiac resynchronization therapy, and device implantation (eg, implantable cardioverter–defibrillators and mechanical circulatory support devices). However, these patients still have heart failure and the use of and discontinuation of these devices need to be considered,[13] because continued use of devices may not prolong life, but instead prolong dying.[32] A more realistic and updated model of the heart failure illness trajectory is shown in **Fig. 4**.

Failure to Have the Conversation

A second reason why palliative care is not offered is the lack of conversation about advance care planning, advance directives, and goals of care as the patient moves through the heart failure trajectory.[5,7] Typical conversations between health care

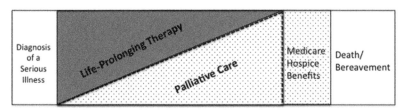

Fig. 1. Typical model of palliative care. (*Adapted from* National Consensus Project. Clinical practice guidelines for quality palliative care. 2nd edition. Pittsburgh (PA): National Consensus Project for Quality Palliative Care; 2009.)

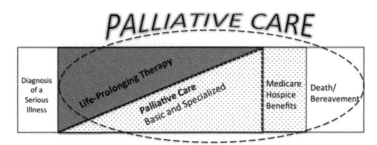

Fig. 2. Model of palliative care as an encompassing philosophy of care. (*Adapted from* National Consensus Project. Clinical practice guidelines for quality palliative care. 2nd edition. Pittsburgh (PA): National Consensus Project for Quality Palliative Care; 2009.)

providers and patients focus on disease management and not end-of-life discussions. As a result, many patients do not even understand the terminality of heart failure.[33] As stated, health care providers are not comfortable with initiating these conversations, but once initiated, many patients want to continue the discussion.[6,7] Providers may need additional support and skills training to learn how to begin these conversations without worrying about taking away hope or fearing patients may perceive the conversations as being abandoned by the provider.[25]

Lack of Understanding of Palliative Care as an Overarching Philosophy Encompassing Hospice

Health care providers do not always have a clear understanding of palliative care and many cannot differentiate palliative care from hospice; thus, patients and their families are not offered these much-needed services.[23,24] Additionally, providers do not always realize that providing palliative care or referring a patient and family to the specialized service is not prognosis dependent and is part of life-prolonging treatment.[25] Without a clear understanding of palliative care, there is a fear of offering services too early owing to the belief that this service should be reserved for those near death.[4] As discussed, palliative care encompasses care provided through the whole heart failure illness trajectory, from diagnosis to death and bereavement. The intensity of palliative care and the type and providers of palliative care (eg, basic vs specialized) may change throughout the trajectory, as depicted by the curved line in **Fig. 5**.

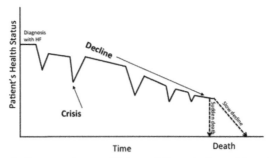

Fig. 3. Typical chronic disease trajectory. HF, heart failure. (*Adapted from* Committee on care at the end of life, Field MJ, Cassel CK, editors. Approaching death: improving care at the end of life. Washington, DC: National Academy Press; 1997.)

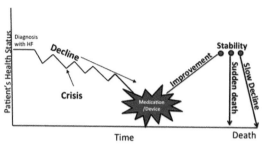

Fig. 4. Heart failure (HF) disease trajectory.

Lack of Available Services/Teams

Although there is consensus that palliative care should be offered from the time of diagnosis for patients with a serious life-limiting illness, the availability of specialized teams limits these services, many times to patients approaching the end of life.[34] Thus, a gap exists between what specialized palliative care teams are able to offer and the needs of all palliative care hospitalized patients.[29] The use of basic palliative care, provided by non–palliative care–certified providers could meet this need; however, many health care providers feel ill-equipped to provide these services and the resources to assist them are not readily available.[35] In many areas of the country, there are limited specialty services and a lack of education for the provision of basic palliative care.[28]

An additional reason why services are not used, is related to patients and/or their family caregivers refusing to accept services.[36] Use of services, including hospice, is influenced by cultural and religious attitudes, as well as patient preferences.[17] Patients and their family caregivers also may not understand the terminality of heart failure, with the belief that patient always got better before.[2,24,26,33,37,38]

BASIC PALLIATIVE CARE FOR HEART FAILURE

Nurses are the bridge to palliative care services for patients with heart failure. There are many aspects of nursing care that are in line with basic palliative care interventions. By understanding what staff nurses, advanced practice nurses, and other health care providers can provide on a daily basis, specialized services can be reserved for when the patients' needs are too complex for basic palliative care.[29] Patients and their families face numerous challenges when living with advanced heart failure, which include physiologic, psychological/emotional, functional, social, and financial concerns.[39] Families encounter additional challenges because their needs are not

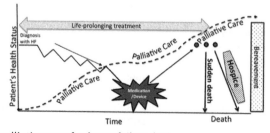

Fig. 5. Model of palliative care for heart failure (HF).

always assessed and their issues are not addressed, but are at risk for poor health outcomes and depression, especially when the patient is critically ill.[40] Basic palliative care can help to address some of these concerns and challenges with the patient's and family's goals for care.[25]

Goodlin[41] provides a comprehensive description of care for patients with heart failure that varies based on the New York Heart Association's functional status classification and illness severity. Descriptions are given for general heart failure care (diagnosis, medications, and plans/goals of care) and supportive care, which includes communication, education, psychosocial or spiritual issues, and symptom management. The supportive care is part of basic palliative care that can be offered by all nurses and other non–palliative care–certified health care providers. The principles of palliative care for heart failure include managing burdensome symptoms that decrease functioning and quality of life and supportive care to address other issues.[10] Included throughout the provision of palliative care is the continual conversation about goals of care, throughout the course of the disease and, in particular, as the patient's condition changes and as advanced medical management and devices are discussed and implanted.

There are 4 overarching components of palliative care for patients with heart failure: the patient's physical issues and uncontrolled symptoms, emotional issues, social issues, and spiritual issues.[8] These areas can be addressed through a comprehensive assessment and evaluation, followed by planned interventions to meet the identified needs of the patient. To begin to assess these issues, nurses need to have an open line of communication with the patient and his or her family members. Within this open communication, discussions related to goals of care based on potential treatment options, end-of-life wishes (including advance directives, advance care planning, and device deactivation) can be included in the conversation[8,13] (For a full description discussing goals of care for patients with cardiovascular disease, see Dunlay and Strand 2015[42]). During these encounters, nurses can both communicate with, counsel, and educate the patient and family about heart failure, proposed treatment options, and available supportive services, including financial services.

Patients and their family caregivers may not seem to be distressed emotionally, but really do need time to talk about the challenges they face living with heart failure. The nurse should evaluate the patient and family caregivers' ability to handle the challenges associated with heart failure, assess whether their goals for care match the plan of care, and determine whether the goals for care realistic based on severity of the heart failure. Nursing interventions include spending time talking to the patient and family caregiver, giving advice, explaining the types of available supportive services, explaining where they can get support, and referring to a social worker or chaplain, if needed.

Patients and their caregivers also may not fully understand heart failure and its trajectory and they may need further explanation of the numerous options for heart failure management that they have been presented. The nurse should assess the patient and caregivers' knowledge base, asking them what they understand about the heart failure and the treatment options presented to them. Education is extremely important here. This should include education about heart failure, where to access additional information about heart failure and its treatment options, what to expect as the disease progresses, and answer questions about management options.

Table 1 shows components of basic palliative care and nurses' role in providing palliative care. These components were adapted from the Institute of Medicine's "Dying in America, Improving Quality and Honoring Individual Preferences Near the End of Life"; the American Heart Association/American Stroke Association's

Table 1
Components of palliative care for heart failure

Component	Rationale	Nursing Care	Nursing Intervention
Physical: Symptom management	Uncontrolled symptoms result in a decreased quality of life and additional burden on the patient and the family caregiver.	Assess for uncontrolled symptoms, such as pain, shortness of breath.	Treat via standing orders, discuss with heart failure team if symptoms persist. Consider referral to specialized palliative care, if uncontrollable.
Emotional issues	Depression is common in heart failure,[10] as is emotional distress.	Assess for depression and emotional distress.	Discuss suspected depression with the health care team and family caregiver. Spend time with the patient, allowing time to verbalize feelings/concerns.
Social/family issues	Having a chronic, life-limiting illness can place a strain on families. Patients may not be able to perform activities of daily living without assistance and at some point, may need continuous assistance.	Assess the family/social situation to determine what issues are present and the ability of the family to care for the patient at home.	Education about caring for the patient at home may ease some of the tension (eg, how to use a weekly organizer for medications); at other times, a referral may be needed for financial or social services.
Spiritual issues	Serious life-limiting illnesses can have a spiritual/religious component, even for individuals who do not consider themselves "religious."	Discuss their beliefs with the patient and family caregiver.	Refer the patient and/or caregiver to the chaplain, if needed.
End-of-life care	As patients transition to end of life, many of these issues need to be addressed; cultural and ethical aspects of end-of-life care need to be assessed.	Patients and families should be supported through the end-of-life transition and families require additional support through bereavement.	Nurses can support the patient and family through end of life; referral to the specialized palliative team and to hospice is warranted.
Family caregiver assessment	Family caregivers are integral partners in the care of the patient and their well-being is important.	Assessment of family well-being as part of the nursing assessment.	Support the family and provide guidance on managing the patient and taking care of themselves.

"Principles for Palliative Care"[10]; Goodlin's "Palliative Care in Congestive Heart Failure"[41]; the International Association for Hospice and Palliative Care (OAHPC), "IAHPC List of Essential Practice in Palliative Care"[43]; and Pastor and Moore's "Uncertainties of the Heart, Palliative Care and Adult Heart Failure."[44] In addition to the 4 components of palliative care (physical, emotional, social, and spiritual), end-of-life care and family caregiver assessment are discussed. Furthermore, the National Consensus Project for the Advancement of Palliative Care[19] lists other domains that need to be considered. These include the cultural aspects of care and end-of-life decisions and the ethical and legal aspects of care.

According to the IOM report, "frequent assessment of the patient's *physical, emotional, social, and spiritual* well-being"[8(pS-7)] must be undertaken. This is imperative because a patient's condition changes continually (either declining or improving) and new medical interventions are proposed. These assessments, which are part of routine nursing care, need to be updated and ongoing to reflect accurately the changing needs of the patient and family caregiver. Staff nurses and advanced practice nurses are able to manage many of the patient and caregiver's needs. However, if there are issues that are unmanageable, they should be discussed with the health care team, and ultimately referred to the specialized palliative care team, when necessary.

FUTURE DIRECTION OF PALLIATIVE CARE IN HEART FAILURE

Palliative care plays an important role in addressing the complex needs of patients and families living with heart failure, a serious life-limiting illness. All nurses should be advocates for patients with heart failure and their family caregivers and be prepared to initiate specialized palliative care consults for all patients with advanced heart failure. However, the role of nursing does not end with this consultation. Basic palliative care provided by nurses must continue and nurses must be active members of the interdisciplinary team caring for the patient and family caregiver. As seen in **Fig. 2**, palliative care is an overarching philosophy that begins with the diagnosis of a serious, life-limiting illness and continues through hospice and bereavement. Caring for heart failure patients and their families is even more complex than depicted in **Fig. 5**, and requires nurses, as part of the interdisciplinary health care team, to be continually assessing the ever-changing needs of these patients and families.

Areas for future improvement can be addressed through research and in clinical practice, and with education. It is known that in-patient specialized palliative care consultations have been found to improve outcomes such as symptom burden, depression, and quality of life as compared with routine care.[45] What has not been studied is whether these improved outcomes would be similar with basic palliative care provided by staff nurses, advanced practice nurses, and non–palliative care–certified cardiologists. The problem is that many nonspecialized health care providers, including nurses, do not feel comfortable providing basic palliative care and are even less comfortable starting the conversation about advance care planning, goal setting, and other end-of-life topics. Education on these areas needs to be strengthened in the curriculum for nursing students and medical students. It also must be included in hospital orientation for all health care providers and part of mandatory continuing education for all providers.

We know that nurses have an important role in supporting, counseling, and educating patients and their family caregivers as they transition through the heart failure trajectory. Nurses are optimally positioned to promote the recommendations of the IOM report advocating for the inclusion of palliative care early in the illness trajectory—with timely referrals to specialized services and hospice.[46] Through the use of basic and specialized palliative care, nurses can address the holistic needs of both patients and families living with a serious life-limiting illness such as heart failure while improving outcomes and quality of life through the heart failure illness trajectory.

REFERENCES

1. Mozaffarian D, Benjamin EJ, Go AS, et al. Heart disease and stroke statistics–2015 update: a report from the American Heart Association. Circulation 2015; 131(4):e29–322.
2. Chen-Scarabelli C, Saravolatz L, Hirsh B, et al. Dilemmas in end-stage heart failure. J Geriatr Cardiol 2015;12(1):57–65.
3. Krumholz HM, Lin Z, Keenan PS, et al. Relationship between hospital readmission and mortality rates for patients hospitalized with acute myocardial infarction, heart failure, or pneumonia. JAMA 2013;309(6):587–93.
4. Kavalieratos D, Mitchell EM, Carey TS, et al. "Not the 'grim reaper service'": an assessment of provider knowledge, attitudes, and perceptions regarding palliative care referral barriers in heart failure. J Am Heart Assoc 2014;3(1):e000544.
5. Barclay S, Momen N, Case-Upton S, et al. End-of-life care conversations with heart failure patients: a systematic literature review and narrative synthesis. Br J Gen Pract 2011;61(582):e49–62.
6. Gadoud A, Jenkins SM, Hogg KJ. Palliative care for people with heart failure: summary of current evidence and future direction. Palliat Med 2013;27(9):822–8.
7. Beattie JM. Palliative care for heart failure: challenges and opportunities. Eur J Cardiovasc Nurs 2014;13(2):102–4.
8. Institute of Medicine (IOM). Dying in America: improving quality and honoring individual preferences near the end of life. Washington, DC: The National Academies Press; 2014.
9. Butler J, Binney Z, Kalogeropoulos A, et al. Advance directives among hospitalized patients with heart failure. JACC Heart Fail 2015;3(2):112–21.
10. Braun LT, American Heart Association's Advocacy Coordinating Committee. American Heart Association/American Stroke Association Principles for Palliative Care. 2013.
11. Dunlay SM, Redfield MM, Jiang R, et al. Care in the last year of life for community patients with heart failure. Circ Heart Fail 2015;8(3):489–96.
12. Lemond L, Allen LA. Palliative care and hospice in advanced heart failure. Prog Cardiovasc Dis 2011;54(2):168–78.
13. Whellan DJ, Goodlin SJ, Dickinson MG, et al. End-of-life care in patients with heart failure. J Card Fail 2014;20(2):121–34.
14. Bakitas M, Macmartin M, Trzepkowski K, et al. Palliative care consultations for heart failure patients: how many, when, and why? J Card Fail 2013;19(3):193–201.
15. Adler ED, Goldfinger JZ, Kalman J, et al. Palliative care in the treatment of advanced heart failure. Circulation 2009;120(25):2597–606.
16. National Hospice and Palliative Care Organization (NHPCO). NHPCO's facts and figures: hospice care in America 2013 Edition. Alexandria (VA): NHCPO; 2013. p. 1–18.
17. Whellan DJ, Cox M, Hernandez AF, et al. Utilization of hospice and predicted mortality risk among older patients hospitalized with heart failure: findings from GWTG-HF. J Card Fail 2012;18(6):471–7.
18. Caffrey C, Sengupta M, Moss A, et al. Home health care and discharged hospice care patients: United States, 2000 and 2007. National Health Statistics reports; no 38. Hyattsville (MD): National Center for Health Statistics; 2011.

19. National Consensus Project. Clinical practice guidelines for quality palliative care. 2nd edition. Pittsburgh (PA): National Consensus Project for Quality Palliative Care; 2009.

20. WHO. WHO Definition of Palliative Care. 2015. Available at: www.who.int/cancer/palliative/definition/en/. Accessed March 20, 2015.

21. National Quality Forum (NQF). A national framework and preferred practices for palliative and hospice care quality: a consensus report. Washington, DC: NQF; 2006.

22. Kitko L, Hupcey JE, Palese M. Palliative care services during terminal hospitalization: stage D heart failure patients. In Heart Failure Society of America, 2014 Scientific Assembly. Las Vegas (NV), September 16, 2014.

23. Gelfman LP, Kalman J, Goldstein NE. Engaging heart failure clinicians to increase palliative care referrals: overcoming barriers, improving techniques. J Palliat Med 2014;17(7):753–60.

24. Hupcey JE, Penrod J, Fogg J. Heart failure and palliative care: implications in practice. J Palliat Med 2009;12(6):531–6.

25. Lindvall C, Hultman TD, Jackson VA. Overcoming the barriers to palliative care referral for patients with advanced heart failure. J Am Heart Assoc 2014;3(1): e000742.

26. Metzger M, Norton SA, Quinn JR, et al. Patient and family members' perceptions of palliative care in heart failure. Heart Lung 2013;42(2):112–9.

27. Metzger M, Norton SA, Quinn JR, et al. "That don't work for me": patients' and family members' perspectives on palliative care and hospice in late-stage heart failure. J Hosp Palliat Nurs 2013;15(3):177–82.

28. Fink RM, Oman KS, Youngwerth J, et al. A palliative care needs assessment of rural hospitals. J Palliat Med 2013;16(6):638–44.

29. Weissman DE, Meier DE. Identifying patients in need of a palliative care assessment in the hospital setting: a consensus report from the Center to Advance Palliative Care. J Palliat Med 2011;14(1):17–23.

30. Kheirbek RE, Alemi F, Citron BA, et al. Trajectory of illness for patients with congestive heart failure. J Palliat Med 2013;16(5):478–84.

31. Hupcey JE, Penrod J, Fenstermacher K. A model of palliative care for heart failure. Am J Hosp Palliat Care 2009;26(5):399–404.

32. Sobanski P, Jaarsma T, Krajnik M. End-of-life matters in chronic heart failure patients. Curr Opin Support Palliat Care 2014;8(4):364–70.

33. Kitko L, Hupcey JE. Patients' perceptions of illness severity in advanced heart failure in Heart failure 2015. Seville (Spain): The Heart Failure Association of the European Society of Cardiology; 2015.

34. Hupcey JE, Kitko L. Health policy implications: outpatient palliative care for heart failure. In American Academy of Nursing 40th Annual Meeting and Conference. Washington DC, October, 2013.

35. Fitzsimons D, Mullan D, Wilson JS, et al. The challenge of patients' unmet palliative care needs in the final stages of chronic illness. Palliat Med 2007;21(4):313–22.

36. Hupcey JE, Kitko L. Perceptions and utilization of palliative care services for HF patients at end of life. In Eastern Nursing Research Society, 27th Annual Scientific Session. Washington, DC, April 17, 2015.

37. Hermani S, Letizia M. Providing palliative care in end-stage heart failure. J Hosp Palliat Nurs 2008;10(2):100–5.

38. Hupcey JE, Kitko L. The troubled water under the bridge: lack of palliative care referrals for heart failure. In European Association for Palliative Care, 14th World Congress. Copenhagen (Denmark), May 8, 2015.

39. Albert NM, Paul S, Murray M. Complexities of care for patients and families living with advanced cardiovascular diseases: overview. J Cardiovasc Nurs 2012;27(2):103–13.
40. Haines KJ, Denehy L, Skinner EH, et al. Psychosocial outcomes in informal caregivers of the critically ill: a systematic review. Crit Care Med 2015;43(5):1112–20.
41. Goodlin SJ. Palliative care in congestive heart failure. J Am Coll Cardiol 2009;54(5):386–96.
42. Dunlay MS, Strand JJ. How-to discuss goals of care with patients. Trends Cardiovasc Med 2015. [Epub ahead of print].
43. IAHPC. IAHPC list of essential practice in palliative care. 2013. Available at: www.hospicecare.com. Accessed March 30, 2015.
44. Pastor DK, Moore G. Uncertainties of the heart palliative care and adult heart failure. Home Healthc Nurse 2013;31(1):29–36.
45. Sidebottom AC, Jorgenson A, Richards H, et al. Inpatient palliative care for patients with acute heart failure: outcomes from a randomized trial. J Palliat Med 2015;18(2):134–42.
46. Meghani SH, Hinds PS. Policy brief: the Institute of Medicine report Dying in America: improving quality and honoring individual preferences near the end of life. Nurs Outlook 2015;63(1):51–9.

United States Postal Service

Statement of Ownership, Management, and Circulation
(All Periodicals Publications Except Requestor Publications)

1. Publication Title	2. Publication Number	3. Filing Date
Critical Care Nursing Clinics of North America	0 0 6 - 2 7 3	9/18/15

4. Issue Frequency	5. Number of Issues Published Annually	6. Annual Subscription Price
Mar, Jun, Sep, Dec	4	$150.00

7. Complete Mailing Address of Known Office of Publication (Not printer) (Street, city, county, state, and ZIP+4®)

Elsevier Inc.
360 Park Avenue South
New York, NY 10010-1710

Contact Person: Stephen R. Bushing
Telephone (Include area code): 215-239-3688

8. Complete Mailing Address of Headquarters or General Business Office of Publisher (Not printer)

Elsevier Inc., 360 Park Avenue South, New York, NY 10010-1710

9. Full Names and Complete Mailing Addresses of Publisher, Editor, and Managing Editor (Do not leave blank)

Publisher (Name and complete mailing address)

Linda Belfus, Elsevier Inc., 1600 John F. Kennedy Blvd., Suite 1800, Philadelphia, PA 19103

Editor (Name and complete mailing address)

Kerry Holland, Elsevier Inc., 1600 John F. Kennedy Blvd., Suite 1800, Philadelphia, PA 19103-2899

Managing Editor (Name and complete mailing address)

Adrianne Brigido, Elsevier Inc., 1600 John F. Kennedy Blvd., Suite 1800, Philadelphia, PA 19103-2899

10. Owner (Do not leave blank. If the publication is owned by a corporation, give the name and address of the corporation immediately followed by the names and addresses of all stockholders owning or holding 1 percent or more of the total amount of stock. If not owned by a corporation, give the names and addresses of the individual owners. If owned by a partnership or other unincorporated firm, give its name and address as well as those of each individual owner. If the publication is published by a nonprofit organization, give its name and address.)

Full Name	Complete Mailing Address
Wholly owned subsidiary of	1600 John F. Kennedy Blvd, Ste. 1800
Reed/Elsevier, US holdings	Philadelphia, PA 19103-2899

11. Known Bondholders, Mortgagees, and Other Security Holders Owning or Holding 1 Percent or More of Total Amount of Bonds, Mortgages, or Other Securities. If none, check box. ☑ None

Full Name	Complete Mailing Address
N/A	

12. Tax Status (For completion by nonprofit organizations authorized to mail at nonprofit rates) (Check one)
The purpose, function, and nonprofit status of this organization and the exempt status for federal income tax purposes:
☐ Has Not Changed During Preceding 12 Months
☐ Has Changed During Preceding 12 Months (Publisher must submit explanation of change with this statement)

13. Publication Title	14. Issue Date for Circulation Data Below
Critical Care Nursing Clinics of North America	September 2015

15. Extent and Nature of Circulation			Average No. Copies Each Issue During Preceding 12 Months	No. Copies of Single Issue Published Nearest to Filing Date
a. Total Number of Copies (Net press run)			396	327
b. Legitimate Paid and Or Requested Distribution (By Mail and Outside the Mail)	(1)	Mailed Outside County Paid/Requested Mail Subscriptions stated on PS Form 3541. (Include paid distribution above nominal rate, advertiser's proof copies and exchange copies)	229	185
	(2)	Mailed In-County Paid/Requested Mail Subscriptions stated on PS Form 3541. (Include paid distribution above nominal rate, advertiser's proof copies and exchange copies)		
	(3)	Paid Distribution Outside the Mails Including Sales Through Dealers And Carriers, Street Vendors, Counter Sales, and Other Paid Distribution Outside USPS®	59	57
	(4)	Paid Distribution by Other Classes of Mail Through the USPS (e.g. First-Class Mail®)		
c. Total Paid or Requested Circulation (Sum of 15b (1), (2), (3), and (4))			288	242
d. Free or Nominal Rate Distribution (By Mail and Outside the Mail)	(1)	Free or Nominal Rate Outside-County Copies included on PS Form 3541	41	43
	(2)	Free or Nominal Rate In-County Copies included on PS Form 3541		
	(3)	Free or Nominal Rate Copies mailed at Other classes Through the USPS (e.g. First-Class Mail®)		
	(4)	Free or Nominal Rate Distribution Outside the Mail (Carriers or Other means)		
e. Total Nonrequested Distribution (Sum of 15d (1), (2), (3) and (4))			41	43
f. Total Distribution (Sum of 15c and 15e)			329	285
g. Copies not Distributed (See instructions to publishers #4 (page #3))			67	42
h. Total (Sum of 15f and g)			396	327
i. Percent Paid and/or Requested Circulation (15c divided by 15f times 100)			87.54%	84.91%

* If you are claiming electronic copies go to line 16 on page 3. If you are not claiming Electronic copies, skip to line 17 on page 3

16. Electronic Copy Circulation	Average No. Copies Each Issue During Preceding 12 Months	No. Copies of Single Issue Published Nearest to Filing Date
a. Paid Electronic Copies		
b. Total paid Print Copies (Line 15c) + Paid Electronic copies (Line 16a)		
c. Total Print Distribution (Line 15f) + Paid Electronic Copies (Line 16a)		
d. Percent Paid (Both Print & Electronic copies) (16b divided by 16c X 100)		

☐ I certify that 50% of all my distributed copies (electronic and print) are paid above a nominal price

17. Publication of Statement of Ownership
☑ If the publication is a general publication, publication of this statement is required Will be printed in the December 2015 issue of this publication

18. Signature and Title of Editor, Publisher, Business Manager, or Owner

Stephen R. Bushing

Stephen R. Bushing – Inventory Distribution Coordinator

Date: September 18, 2015

I certify that all information furnished on this form is true and complete. I understand that anyone who furnishes false or misleading information on this form or who omits material or information requested on the form may be subject to criminal sanctions (including fines and imprisonment) and/or civil sanctions (including civil penalties).

PS Form **3526**, July 2014 (Page 2 of 3)

Printed and bound by CPI Group (UK) Ltd, Croydon, CR0 4YY

03/10/2024

01040487-0018